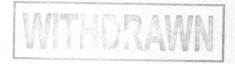

Welfare and Policy
Research Agendas and Issues

Edited by
Neil Lunt
Douglas Coyle

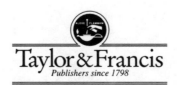

Taylor & Francis
Publishers since 1798

UK   Taylor & Francis Ltd, 1 Gunpowder Square, London EC4A 3DE
USA   Taylor & Francis Inc., 1900 Frost Road, Suite 101, Bristol, PA 19007

First published 1996

Library catalogue record for this book is available from the British Library

ISBN 0 7484 0401 5
ISBN 0 7484 0402 3 (pbk)

Library of Congress Cataloging-in-Publication Data are available on request

Cover design by Hybert Design & Type.

Typeset in 10/12 pt Times
by Solidus (Bristol) Limited

Printed in Great Britain by SRP Ltd, Exeter

Contents

Section II: New Issues

Acknowledgments

This book owes much to discussions at the Institute for Research in the Social Sciences (IRISS) Conference held at the University of York in the Autumn of 1994. The editors would like to thank Peter McLaverty, Jan Sørenson and Alex Watt who helped organize the conference and all those who participated.

Thanks are also due to those involved in the preparation of this volume. Keith Hartley provided practical support. Jan Sørenson, Carl Thompson, David Buck, Peter Kemp and Ken Wright made helpful comments on earlier drafts of chapters. Our thanks also go to Barbara Dodds who organized the final text with precision and Kate Green for her detailed reading of all contributions. Comfort Jegede and Fiona Kinghorn at Taylor & Francis offered encouragement and assistance throughout our endeavours.

Finally, we are indebted to Anne Corden. She gave advice throughout the planning and delivery of this project; read contributions; and made numerous invaluable suggestions. Our only regret is that we did not listen to her nearly enough.

Preface

This book arose from the Fourth IRISS Conference which took place at Kings Manor, York in the Autumn of 1994. IRISS – The Institute for Research in the Social Sciences – is the largest group of social scientists working in the UK in related policy fields: social and health care; social work; health economics; social security and living standards; and housing. It draws together contributions including sociology; public administration; political philosophy; economics; and management science.

The IRISS Conference provides an opportunity for researchers working across these policy fields and disciplines to meet together to discuss their work. The forum offers an occasion for colleagues in related disciplines working around similar issues to explore methodologies, share results and highlight emergent themes.

The Conference is an extremely fruitful event, whose strength lies in the fact that discussions begun there are taken forward and developed. Each IRISS Conference adopts a theme wide enough to ensure that all of its disciplines can be included in the debates. The theme of this year's conference centred around issues of public and private welfare. Each conference results in a published volume of papers that illustrates themes, perspectives and issues advanced by participants, and subsequently developed. A wealth of publications has resulted from past years' conferences[1].

Following in this tradition, *Welfare and Policy* is a selection of contributions based around welfare issues, demonstrating the scope of interests, approaches and methodologies. In so doing it allows us to link underlying themes and developments from comparative perspectives. It is not in any way meant as a text. Textbooks dwell upon the past, are preoccupied with terms and do not address policy and practice. In contrast this volume looks forward, offering commentary on recent policy initiatives, exploring the implications of policy measures and illuminating future agendas. Research contributes to an awareness of the choices we make and the conceptual and methodological boundaries within which we work. Even if questions are not answered definitively we may, through debate and discussion, come closer to asking some of the right ones.

In assembling this collection we have been struck by the similarities between the chapters and an underlying theme of the recent Report of the Commission on Social Justice (1994)[2] – that welfare itself is a curious mixture of both old and new. The Commission on Social Justice was an independent body, set up by the late John Smith, with a view to developing a 'practical vision of economic and social reform for the next century'. The Commission began its work in 1992, the fiftieth anniversary of the Beveridge Report, *Social Insurance and Allied Services*[3], the cornerstone of the UK welfare state. In laying out an agenda for the next century, the Commission refers to the aim of eliminating the social evils initially identified by Beveridge.

The first part of this book discusses what Beveridge 50 years ago identified as the social evils of *disease, squalor* and *want*. Concerns about what Beveridge identified as *disease* have shifted in the 1990s to an emphasis on the maintenance of health. IRISS has a large programme of work on health economics and the management of health administration. It is from this discipline that David Mayston offers an assessment of NHS reforms; debating motives underlying the recent changes and questioning why so little of the reforms were established on research-based evidence. Systems he suggests, just as with the introduction of individual drugs, need to be thought through before being put into action. Significant factors contributing to good health lie outside the structural reforms identified in the first chapter. The Centre for Health Economics at York has developed an extensive programme on the effects of alcohol consumption for example. David Buck, Christine Godfrey and Gerald Richardson enter the domain of fiscal incentives and explore the relationship between price, tax and consumption of alcohol. Their chapter points to the need to consider both individual and social costs of alcohol consumption. Both chapters remind us that detailed empirical work has an important role in highlighting gaps in existing data sources.

As the Commission on Social Justice acknowledged, what Beveridge identified as *squalor* has, in the context of 1990s debates, broadened to become the issue of what constitutes a safe environment. Despite the term *squalor* having become unfashionable, it still seems however, the most appropriate term for describing the topic of the next chapter. Homelessness has become one of the most visible welfare agendas of the 1990s. The chapter from Peter McLaverty, David Rhodes and Hilary Third, in bringing together research evidence, offers an assessment of the likely outcome of measures aimed at addressing homelessness. Solutions aimed at eliminating the role of the public sector have gained favour in many areas of public life; this chapter suggests its prospects in the area of homelessness are not particularly promising. The following chapter on drug abuse illustrates that discussions around what constitutes a safe environment take different forms over time. The chapter by Christine Godfrey and Matthew Sutton discusses the treatment of drug problems, and outlines the effects of a particular treatment – that of methadone maintenance programmes – on both individuals and society. Importantly, the chapter reminds us that research cannot avoid taking decisions about the relative trade-offs of drug abuse and interventions.

A further issue identified by Beveridge centred around what he termed *want*. However, in current debates language has shifted and we no longer talk about *want*: concern and discussion centre on how to measure *need*, and how to meet needs. In the light of this it would seem time for a critical re-assessment of the means-test as a measurement of financial needs. Tony Eardley explores the means-test for social assistance; initially advanced as a residual policy measure, means-testing now occupies a central role in our social security system. Drawing upon comparative international evidence, the chapter places UK policy in a wider context, raising debates around the workings of the means-test. Budgetary constraints inevitably exist on the extent to which any needs can be met. Neil Lunt, Russell Mannion and Peter Smith in their chapter on community care finance explore the meeting of needs in an area which – as a result of demographic, ideological and policy changes – has become one of the most pressing welfare agendas for the 1990s. The chapter explores the relationship between funding, eligibility criteria and boundaries with services such as the NHS; and illustrates that welfare is inclined not to fit easily into predetermined categories.

The final chapter in the section is by John Horton and moves us from technical details of policy implementation to a reflection on the values underlying it, noting: 'empirical research no matter how well devised and conducted, cannot answer all our questions about social policies'. In exhorting us to broaden our conception of community care and enquire into its wider meaning, he asks some searching questions about the relationship between individuals and communities.

Unlike the collection of papers in the first section, which reflected the recycling of welfare agendas, albeit under the cover of different terms; those in the second section remind us that, as social scientists, we are also faced with rapidly unfolding agendas: policy reforms; demographic shifts; structural changes; and ideological developments all impact directly on welfare, forming agendas and issues that researchers must both develop and follow.

The role of the market has been a dominant feature of 1990s welfare discourse, and Roy Sainsbury and Steven Kennedy examine the place of the market *vis-à-vis* social security administration. Their chapter explores and appraises how markets operate and unfold in this newer area. Adopting the market as a policy area, as Sainsbury and Kennedy note, brings into focus aspects of consumerism and accountability. Jane Lightfoot in her chapter outlines how changes in health policy have contributed to a rethinking of the notion of accountability. Accountability, she argues, must explore the domain of professional accountability if it is to offer a full account. The chapter by Karl Atkin offers the fundamental challenge to create a welfare system that is sensitive to the needs of all groups in society. The discipline of social policy and most policy researchers, Atkin argues, have remained indifferent to the impact of race on welfare agendas; and his chapter offers some analytical categories to assist researchers in tackling the issues raised.

John Ditch in his chapter reminds us that the political environment within which policy develops cannot be neglected; and that we must remember pressures helping to shape current and future agendas are both external and internal. Although *Welfare and Policy* addresses UK policy, research cannot remain insular in relation to wider developments. John Ditch's chapter explores the convergence of European social policy in relation to social protection. It outlines the likely prospects for the UK in relation to future European developments.

Just as the chapter by John Ditch reminds us that welfare policy develops within a wider political and institutional environment, the final chapter by Neil Small illustrates that research activity is itself located within an ideological, methodological, and institutional framework. When we consider approaches to welfare he suggests that we assess the blend of values, empiricism, and theory that cover all social sciences.

Indeed, to develop a point made by Neil Small, these chapters, as a combination of disciplines and policy areas, follow no single disciplinary style. Discourse is not only what we say; it is how we say it, relating to the usage of terms and the flow of language. When bringing together the disciplines of economics, sociology and social policy we cannot expect writers to cut themselves adrift from their theoretical roots. Here we return to our starting point: that there is richness to be gained through communication across disciplines and policy fields by researchers approaching agendas and issues with their own distinctive expertise.

Neil Lunt
Douglas Coyle
July 1995

Notes

1   Publications from three previous IRISS Conferences are:
    BALDWIN, S., GODFREY, C. and PROPPER, C. (Eds) (1990) *Quality of Life: Perspectives and Policies*, London: Routledge.
    HUTTON, J., HUTTON, S., PINCH, T. and SHEILL, A. (Eds) (1991) *Dependency to Enterprise*, London: Routledge.
    CORDEN, A., ROBERTSON, E. and TOLLEY, K. (Eds) (1992) *Meeting Needs in an Affluent Society*, Aldershot: Avebury.
2   COMMISSION ON SOCIAL JUSTICE (1994) *Strategies for National Renewal*, Report of the Commission on Social Justice, London: Vintage.
3   BEVERIDGE, W. (1942) *Social Insurance and Allied Services*, Cmnd 6404, London: HMSO.

Old Agendas

Chapter 1

Health Care Reform: A Study in Imperfect Information

David Mayston

Introduction

With so many changes taking place in the NHS and in other health care systems around the world (Organisation for Economic Cooperation Development, 1992, 1994), these are interesting times for the study of health care systems. Interest in the changes being made to health care systems comes not only from academics and professionals involved in the health care field, but also from potential consumers of health care. The interest for consumers extends not only to whether it is possible to improve the operation of health care systems, but also to whether there is any risk of the system actually functioning less well as a result of the proposed changes. Both aversion to the risk of things going wrong and an assessment of the size of the risks involved are natural concerns of potential consumers of health care.

As academic analysts, we may recall that 'May you live in interesting times' was indeed an ancient Chinese curse. An interesting medical condition is not the same thing as a healthy medical condition. Individual consumers naturally dislike potentially risky interventions into their personal biological systems, however interesting it may be for the medics involved. The consumers of health care are only likely to willingly accept such risks if they believe that the case for such interventions has been carefully assessed in advance.

Before attempting any final conclusions on matters medical or otherwise, academics and scientists seek to deploy the processes of free-ranging investigation, theoretical probing, careful empirical testing and the open detailed discussion of the results. These processes are intended not just to be interesting in themselves. They are aimed principally at minimizing the risk of false conclusions being drawn. In the case of the prescription of drugs, the consequences for individual patients of false conclusions being drawn can indeed be dire. The process of careful scientific testing is therefore deployed on a regular basis, before the introduction of new drugs is permitted, as part of a rigorous system the Government itself lays down.

The Politics of Imperfect Information

In the case of health care reform, the prescribed reforms affect not just individual patients but rather entire populations of the countries involved. However, the principal driving force for the reforms has often not been one of careful scientific endeavour. Instead it has tended, in the UK at least, to be one of political fervour. Within the vocabulary of conviction politics and ideological certainties that have motivated many health care reforms, *risk* is a four-letter word that the vocabulary would rather not embrace. The careful scientific testing of underlying hypo-theses, on the basis of open discussion and controlled experimentation in order to minimize risk, would merely have served to delay the political imperatives that came to drive the NHS Reforms of Margaret Thatcher. The NHS Review that drew up the Reforms was itself conceived and developed in secret. Its resulting blueprint, *Working for Patients* (Department of Health, 1989), was then announced to a suspecting public as a *fait accompli*, to be implemented without further discussion or testing.

Even where there had been previous experimentation in the NHS, as in the six pilot studies for the earlier Resource Management Initiative (RMI), the conclusions of the evaluation of the pilot studies – that there were no clear benefits from the initiative that outweighed the substantial costs involved (Packwood, Keen and Buxton, 1991) – were overlooked. Instead the RMI was to be implemented nationally across the whole of the NHS hospital sector as part of the NHS Reforms.

Rather than attempting to be an open *scientific* enquiry into how best to improve the functioning of the NHS, the conception and implementation of the NHS Reforms have instead at times seemed more akin to entering the shadowy world of John le Carré. One senses powerful ideological forces to be at work in an underworld of imperfect understanding. These forces operate through well-placed agents who seem at times intent on covert actions designed to subvert an existing functioning empire established decades ago by those with alien intentions. In this shadowy new world, one must look through mirrors to see other mirrors to assess the current state of play in the cold war between opposing ideologies. Even up to the final page doubts exist as to the true motivation and intentions of each participant, and suspicion lingers as to which side some of the main characters are really on.

The apparent defection of the former Head of the London Bureau, in the shape of the former Chief Executive of the NHS, to join the board of the aspiring rival superpower BUPA, after blood-curdling treatment in the dark corridors of power of the Public Accounts Committee (PAC) (1993), simply adds to the twists and turns we have witnessed since the NHS Review was announced. The arrest of one of the advocates of the NHS Reforms, and subsequent conviction on drug charges, even provided one or two of the lurid overtones to the surrounding scene that we have come to expect of a modern novel.

Within the twilight world of le Carré, trust is a scarce commodity that is embraced at one's peril. In the NHS White Paper, however, Trust (though not 'trust') is a word that is embraced frequently and without question. There have been those working in rival empires, such as the Chairman of the British Medical Association and politicians in opposition parties, who have questioned whether Trusts were intended, in effect, to be covert 'sleepers' for the ultimate privatization of the NHS. Given the likely political unpopularity of any overt move towards privatization of the NHS, covert behaviour is perhaps not to be fully discounted. How, though, can one decipher the ultimate intentions of some of those involved?

An examination of the outward and visible signs of NHS Trust letterheads reveals new, strangely NHS-free, designations, such as Scarborough and North East Yorkshire Healthcare (SNEYH). Such name changes, and associated re-organizations, would not be out of line with those that have taken place elsewhere in the public sector ahead of privatization, as in the cases of British Coal, RailTrack and Parcel Force. The letterhead emblem of SNEYH stands five centimetres high, 50 times the one-millimetre height of the designation 'NHS Trust' that appears at the bottom of the page. This is a ratio even greater than can be observed in an identifiable case where intended privatization has already been announced, that of Parcel Force. The emblem of Parcel Force now dominates the sides of its van fleet, with the smaller emblem of Royal Mail ready to be painted out following privatization of Parcel Force, but still accorded a greater relative size than that of 'NHS Trust' on SNEYH's own letterhead. If intelligence involves the putting together of small, seemingly unconnected pieces of information, what is one to conclude from such everyday observations?

The reassuring words 'where there is discord, let there be harmony' of the initiator of the NHS Reforms, Margaret Thatcher, did not accord with the impact of many of her policies outside the health care field. Mrs Thatcher's similar declaration under political pressure that 'the NHS is safe in our hands' was re-enforced by the claimed intention of her NHS White Paper *Working for Patients*, as being to strengthen the NHS. However, to Williams (1990a, p. 178) it seemed:

> ... very odd that a Government which has prided itself on its unswerving pursuit of libertarian ideals and a Prime Minister who has avowed her intention to destroy socialism, should appear to be such a staunch defender and supporter of the only really socialist post-war institution to make a substantial impact on British society and to win the

support of the vast majority of the citizenry. There must be a catch somewhere, or has the leopard really changed its spots?

Several chapters into our le Carré drama, we find the original instigator of the NHS Reforms, Margaret Thatcher, involuntarily removed by a very British coup. The political disadvantages of a high profile assault on the NHS have been noted. The direction of the Reforms has instead become more covert, perhaps gaining a momentum of their own, outside the control of any one political power. The steady shifting of patients out of NHS long-stay care and into *social care*, financed wherever possible by private payments, represents a real, though largely undercover, reduction in the responsibilities of the NHS. Impersonal market forces now deflect attention away from central Government as being responsible for the closure of numerous hospital wards and premises. Dentists are allowed to steadily de-register patients from the NHS in their own quiet and voluntary way, following a Government funding settlement that failed to please them.

The principle of Government ministers devolving responsibility for areas of activity that would otherwise threaten political embarrassment, to more independent 'agents' and 'agencies', has long been a theme of the le Carré world of governmental security services. It is now a key part of Government policy towards more visible public services, such as Her Majesty's Prison Service and the NHS.

More than five years on from the NHS White Paper, and several lengthy chapters after its opening aspirations, the more subtle twists and turns of the NHS Reforms may provoke the reader into wanting to abandon its twisted narrative as being too convoluted to wish to follow any further. However, unlike many spy novels, there is no guarantee in health care systems that good will necessarily prevail at the end of the day. Very adverse outcomes can result for vulnerable groups in society from several of the health care changes that have been made in recent years, if all of the details of the changes are not carefully monitored.

The run down of long-stay beds in the NHS under the *Care in the Community* programme, without sufficient accompanying increases in community resources to provide adequate community care, has adversely affected the welfare of vulnerable individual patients, such as schizophrenics (Palmer, 1994). On a larger scale, the position of 37 million US citizens with little or no access to reasonable health care (Aaron, 1991), despite expenditure of some 13.4 per cent of US Gross Domestic Product (GDP) on health care (Organisation for Economic Cooperation Development, 1993), illustrates that socially desirable, and cost-effective, outcomes are not guaranteed by more market-orientated health care systems. This suggests that if health care reforms are to result in beneficial changes, their proposals must be carefully evaluated, with any associated risks fully appraised and reduced to an acceptable level. The excessive level of risk that was implied by the rapid implementation of the original *Working for Patients* proposal was noted by Williams (1990a, p. 191):

> Unless the time scale of the proposals is changed radically, and the encouragement to expand the private sector is abandoned, and the extra resources put instead into the state sector, I fear that the NHS will be thrown into chaos. But perhaps that is a prospect which everyone does not view with the same dismay as I do.

If we value our health care system, as indeed we must, we cannot afford to throw down the real-life story in which we find ourselves, because of the opaque progress of its plot. We need to understand what is happening on each page. How then can we make sense of our le Carré novel in which agents with mixed motives, and less than pure procedures, work in the shadows for opposing superpowers that each proclaim a shining ideological purity of purpose towards the betterment of mankind? To comprehend this twilight world, we need to understand what is going on at several levels.

The first level is undoubtedly a clash of ideology of the kind Williams (1990a, p. 180) articulated in his original chapter in the York volume *Competition in Health Care*. Egalitarianism and libertarianism offer ideologically different perspectives on the future of the NHS and the nature of health care provision. However, the clash between belief-systems involves not only opposing political ideologies. It also involves strongly-held codes of professional ethics that conflict with the shibboleths of managerial efficiency. Fundamental disagreements are aroused that in part reflect differing value judgements about the nature and relative importance of basic philosophical concepts, such as those of Social Welfare, Freedom, Personal Responsibility, Efficiency, Equity and Professional Responsibility to individual patients and disadvantaged groups.

Such ideological clashes, however, soon progress beyond *value judgements* about individual freedom and the distribution of health care to rich and poor. They extend also to a second level, that of *quasi-factual* beliefs about the relative merits in achieving equity and efficiency of public and private provision, of managerial control compared to professional control, and of greater competition within health care systems. In so doing, these quasi-factual beliefs tend to lock on to idealized descriptions of alternative health care systems and of the role of individuals, groups and control processes within them (see Williams 1990a, p. 181).

The third level, as with the mixed motives of le Carré agents, and perhaps also of their controllers, comes to involve the more sordid subject of money and of how the system actually operates in practice. The shining claims of the outward ideology may here become compromised by more self-serving political interest and by scarcity of resources. There are then pressures to reduce the quality of care, and to deflect resources in the search for professional satisfaction into high technology medicine and away from more routine activities.

Just as the Soviet Union fell considerably short of its bold ideological claims, so too in practice is the actual operation of health care systems likely to diverge from their own idealized claims (see Williams, 1990a, p. 183). Even well-paid NHS consultants may pursue their own financial gain from private practice at the expense of their NHS patients (Audit Commission, 1995; Yates, 1995). Equally, the bold claims of the process of Reform may themselves conceal a more patchy and enigmatic reality in which many old tensions remain unresolved, both in the new Russia and in the new NHS.

Ideology may still nevertheless provide the stated and outward rationale for the system to which functionaries, in positions of managerial power within the system, must pay homage. Rather than encouraging a risk-minimizing strategy of open discussion and free debate on the merits of individual changes, ideology provides many pressures towards conformity in the selection and behaviour of those with such power. The NHS Reforms have included the elimination of more independently minded elected members from NHS health authorities. Their replacements are now vetted and appointed under more covert processes by the Secretary of State. The rights of professional members of staff to make public their firsthand information on the shortcomings of the service are now restricted, with continuing allegations of the attempted suppression or dismissal of 'whistle-blowers' within the NHS. Again there are le Carré-style overtones of a more closed and secretive service to which all agents must yield unquestioning loyalty or be eliminated.

Whatever the outward ideology, the self-interest of those in power in their respective superstates may lead to the adoption of similar techniques for the maintenance of their power. Given the political sensitivity of many issues in the NHS, such as waiting lists, the increasing reliance on the techniques of centralized news management within the NHS (*The Independent*, 25 January 1995) may be a natural extension of a more managed service. Centralized news management enables awkward realities to be massaged into a form more in line with the ideological imperatives and the prevailing world-view, and indeed self-interest, of the political leadership. In contrast, permitting a free-ranging scientific examination and discussion of all available evidence is likely to lead to a questioning of the prevailing doctrines, and by implication a questioning of the legitimacy of the current leadership that has espoused these imperatives.

Rather than pursuing a scientific search for objective evidence, health care reform risks falling back to more tribal behaviour. Magic potions are needed to reinforce the power and authority of the witch doctor, whether from the old tribe of the medical professionals, or from the new tribes of conviction politicians, managers and management consultants. Questioning the efficacy or extent of scientific testing of the prescriptions offered merely threatens to undermine this authority. Determining whether or not the prescriptions offered are really efficacious can similarly become of secondary importance to a more self-interested desire to secure power over territory and resources.

A shifting balance of tribal power over territory and resources has indeed characterized much that has occurred as a result of the NHS Reforms. Within the provider sector, the major shift to date has been the diminution of the territorial power of hospital doctors. Hospital doctors have lost power to the fund-holding GPs through the latter's encroachment into purchasing decisions, and have lost even more power to managers, who have increased both in authority and in numbers with the implementation of the NHS Reforms.

The increasing colonisation of the public sector by those displaying the tribal badges of managerialism and privatization may itself result from underlying tensions and mixed motives (see Kay and Thompson, 1986; Mayston, 1993). Management and information technology consultants come in search of substantial fees, which continual managerial change and re-organization in the NHS help to promote. They have little incentive to question the efficacy and value for money of their own advice and prescriptions. More objective evidence (National Audit Office, 1990, 1992) suggests that there is a significant risk of poor value for money being obtained for the NHS.

Whatever the long-term efficiency-improving properties of privatization, the asset sales and reduced public expenditure that often accompany privatization offer politicians the more immediate sweetening fix of an enhanced cash-flow to relieve their current fiscal problems. Similarly, whatever its long-term impact on efficiency, the devolution of greater responsibility to more autonomous, and less directly publicly accountable, NHS Trusts and Commissions enables politicians themselves to 'pass the parcel' of increasingly difficult decisions, and irksome responsibilities, on to others.

Managers within the NHS in turn find that they can side-step the difficult problem of obtaining cost-reductions without any reduction in the package of care. Instead they are able to resort to more subtle managerial strategies aimed at cost-reduction through cost-shifting. Long-stay elderly patients can be moved quietly out of the NHS and into 'social care', where cost falls outside the NHS budget (see Lunt, Mannion and Smith, Chapter 6 of this volume). Declining quality of care and increasing waiting lists for NHS patients can be transformed into positive management opportunities for greater revenue generation from private pay beds within NHS hospitals. How these tensions resolve themselves within the NHS then forms the content of numerous intricate sub-plots that characterize our shadowy new world.

The Economics of Imperfect Information

The opaque nature of many of the effects of the bold institutional changes that were introduced by the NHS Reforms are confirmed by a recent King's Fund Institute study, *Evaluating the NHS Reforms* (Robinson and Le Grand, 1994). It failed to find any extensive and conclusive evidence on the Reforms' detailed effects on patient care. The main reason for this was the lack of any detailed scientific monitoring of their results. The deliberate political avoidance of detailed monitoring and evaluation, and of controlled experiments, has itself shrouded the impact of Reforms in unnecessary secrecy. The lack of careful scientific monitoring means that it is now very difficult to distinguish between the effects of the changes made by the NHS Reforms, the effects of the increases in NHS funding that the Government resorted to immediately before the 1992 General Election, and the impact of trends (such as increases in the number of day cases) that were in existence before the NHS Review.

Even where there is strong evidence of significant changes in behaviour occurring as a result of the NHS Reforms, the detailed information needed to accurately interpret the impact of these changes on different patient groups is lacking. Thus one major controversial change made by the NHS Reforms was that of the introduction of GP fundholders. A recent study by the Association of Community Health Councils for England and Wales (1994) has found strong evidence that patients of fundholding GPs are receiving better access to NHS health care than patients of non-fundholding GPs. However, the lack of carefully controlled monitoring of such a change leaves unclear how far this superior access is due to an absolute improvement in the efficiency of hospitals responding to the greater competitive power of GP fundholders, and how far it is due instead to the diversion of resources away from the patients of non-fundholding GPs. A similar lack of detailed monitoring of the results of the efficiency measures involved in the pre-Review Cost Improvement Programmes (see Mayston, 1990a) in the NHS led an earlier King's Fund Institute (1989) study to conclude that there was insufficient evidence to support a conclusion that the cost savings had been achieved with no loss in the quality of service provided.

The imperfect nature of many NHS statistics on hospital activity makes them open to potential manipulation by those with imperfect motives. As noted by Seng, Lessof and McKee (1993), activity measures based on the number of Finished Consultant Episodes can be increased simply by transferring patients more frequently between different hospital departments. Similarly, the Cost Weighted Activity Index (CWAI) that forms the overall output indicator (Department of Health, 1994) for the whole Hospital and Community Health Services (HCHS) branch of the NHS may well substantially overstate the national increase in hospital activity that it claims to have achieved. HCHS itself spends some £22.8 billion a year on current and capital expenditure. Some 69.9 per cent of the total cost weighting (i.e. nearly £16 billion) within the CWAI for HCHS is on the single undifferentiated category of 'All inpatient episodes and day cases' (see Mayston, 1994a). Despite the large variation in the relative cost of the many different forms of treatment in this single vast category, they are all counted and added together in units of Finished Consultant Episodes –

unweighted within this single large category by any consideration of variation in complexity or length of stay. In this unweighted form, the policy that has been pursued in the NHS in recent years, of steadily discharging long-stay patients and using the released expenditure to fund many additional day cases, results in a far more dramatic increase in the CWAI, and the reported overall activity measure of NHS hospitals, than if there had been more detailed cost-weighting of the many different forms of treatment that actually exist within the very wide and heterogeneous category of 'all inpatient episodes and day cases'.

The uncertain nature of the package which has been imposed on consumers of the NHS by the initiators of the NHS Reforms stands in contrast to the free-market ideology of many of the Reforms' supporters. Under a free market system, consumers would be given freedom to make their own choice with full information on the nature of the product which they are considering acquiring. The model of supermarket efficiency that led Mrs Thatcher to select Lord Rayner of Marks and Spencer, and Sir Roy Griffiths of Sainsbury's, as Head of the Government's Efficiency Unit and Deputy Chairman of the NHS Management Board respectively, similarly does not accord well with many of the proposals of the NHS Reforms. The centralized control over information technology, marketing and purchasing of standardized products, that appears to enhance the efficiency of both Sainsbury's and Marks and Spencer, contrasts with the increased ability of individual Trusts and health care purchasers to make their own decisions on information technology, marketing and the purchasing of supplies as a result of the NHS Reforms.

As noted above, bold Reforms may well imperfectly resolve longer-standing underlying tensions, and the result may be problems of their own which surface later. An earlier set of managerial reforms that were introduced into the NHS by Mrs Thatcher on the advice of Sir Roy Griffiths in 1983 involved the replacement of the previous NHS ethic of 'consensus management' by the new managerial ethic of a single accountable General Manager for each NHS hospital and health authority. Such a greater concentration of power in the hands of a single General Manager, however, carries the risk of less discussion before managerial decisions are made, and a greater potential risk of managerial mistakes being perpetuated in an unchallenged way. Some ten years after the implementation of the Griffiths reforms, the magnitude of such risks has become apparent. The enhanced power of the Regional General Manager of Wessex Regional Health Authority to pursue his own vision of a Regional Information Strategy Plan (RISP), seemingly unchallenged by his managerial underlings (Public Accounts Committee, 1993), may well have contributed to the waste of some £63 million of NHS resources on the project. This sum included substantial fees paid to a large firm of management and information technology consultants. Following the subsequent investigations by the District Auditor, the RISP project was abandoned, according to the Comptroller and Auditor General, 'without any significant benefit having accrued to the region' (National Audit Office, 1992).

The Comptroller and Auditor General also found 'serious conflicts of interest at a senior level' for some of those involved with the project in the Regional Health Authority who had links with the private sector.

One of the key features of health care itself is *imperfect and asymmetric information*. Potential consumers of health care, i.e. patients, typically possess imperfect information in advance of the provision of health care on their own condition and on the effectiveness and risks of different treatments, and less information than the providers of health care possess. Again this contrasts with a typical supermarket transaction in which the consumer typically buys a familiar product with relatively full knowledge of what it will do for them. Unlike many health care treatments, if an initial supermarket purchase fails to please, the consumer may seek full compensation from the supermarket from any ills that may result from consuming its products. They can also readily and costlessly switch their demand at the next regular supermarket visit.

Once imperfect and asymmetric information is an inherent part of the relationship between participants, private sector markets often involve more problematic outcomes than this simple supermarket scenario. Recent years have seen major difficulties in the Lloyds insurance market due to unanticipated risks being shifted on to under-informed Names. The private pensions industry faces a bill of some £3 billion for compensation as a result of the over-selling of inappropriate policies to under-informed clients. Many private sector auditors now face large lawsuits for their alleged failure to detect and/or fully report on the adverse financial circumstances that existed at companies such as Polly Peck, Maxwell Communications and BCCI prior to their collapse (see Mayston, 1993).

These situations of asymmetric and imperfect information are then ones where the assumptions of the standard theorems of economic theory on the efficiency of competitive markets do not hold. We need to be aware, as Rothschild and Stiglitz (1976) emphasize, that 'some of the most important conclusions of economic theory are not robust to considerations of imperfect information'. In the case of health care, in an attempt to cope with imperfect and asymmetric information, non-market relationships have traditionally developed based upon patients placing their trust in health care professionals to safeguard the patient's best interests. That this trust is not always well placed is emphasized by the imperfect information that health care professionals often themselves possess about the effectiveness of many of the forms of treatment that they routinely prescribe. The trust may also be undermined by scope for professional preference towards more interesting high-technology treatments and over-prescription, rather than for simpler forms of treatment and more cinderella specialisms that may be of greater benefit to large volumes of patients. Once considerations of resource limitations are also introduced, safeguarding the best interests of the patient becomes, moreover, a relativistic term, rather than one of absolute ethical priority.

Information and Effectiveness

One rationalization of the NHS Reforms, or perhaps mid-novel deflection in the shifting agenda, is that the reforms are now less concerned with increased *efficiency* from greater competition in the new internal market. Instead their aim is to seek increased *effectiveness* of the health care delivered, through the separation of the provider-role from that of role of purchasers. Individual health authorities in their new role as purchasers are now able to concentrate exclusively on assessing local health care needs and achieving such effectiveness, instead of also running individual hospitals.

However, apart from some flexing of muscles by a number of fund-holding GPs, this separation has not so far yielded much effect. There are two main reasons for this. The first is that the deepest void in the knowledge base of the NHS lies where the information required for need assessment and priority setting should be. The second is that the provider units entered the labour market first and have tended to hire most of the available talent, so that the more difficult purchasing job was in general left to the less experienced people. Support for the purchasing function has belatedly become a high priority.

Paradoxically, the greatest achievement of the NHS Reforms may come to be a widespread recognition that we do not have the knowledge base needed to make the system work as it is supposed to work. This is not a criticism simply of the new system, but also of the old one. The old system had adapted itself to a style of decision making where professional judgement replaced more systematic information, and where professional solidarity at times replaced public accountability.

Money is usually a key factor in motivating people to act in a system friendly way. However, when it comes to their actual capacity to act in a system friendly way, training and information will be key factors. Unfortunately, the pattern of decentralization conventionally adopted in the NHS has been that clinicians saw themselves as primarily responsible for generating benefits (as defined by themselves); managers for getting work done (using routine measures of process); and finance directors for ensuring that everyone stayed within their budgets. None of them has seen the others' responsibilities as any of their business. The result has been doctors who believe that it is unethical to be cost conscious, managers who think that more must mean better, and finance directors who have had little precise idea of the relationship between costs and clinical activities.

If the new purchasing authorities are to overcome the problems of imperfect and asymmetric information that characterize health care at the individual level, it is essential that purchasing authorities become better informed about the effectiveness of different forms of treatment and expenditures. They will then be better able to act as genuine agents on behalf of patients in their purchasing decisions in a cost-effective way. While the NHS Reforms have devolved healthcare purchasing decisions down to an increasing number of GP fund-holders, we still find cases where GPs themselves continue to prescribe, as a result of ill-informed habits, drugs with potentially adverse side effects, despite the ready availability of less risky and equally effective substitutes.

The contrast between the politically driven, and imperfectly conceived, bold aspirations of the controllers of the NHS Reforms and the murky plight of the under-equipped and under-informed field operatives who must decipher and implement their instructions is emphasized by Opit (1993). In his review of the technical documents issued by the NHS Management Executive to individual NHS purchasers and commissioning authorities, he notes that:

> These technical reports are supposed to give guidance to commissioners. These documents are important both because they may reveal hidden purposes of the NHS Reforms and because they show the political, social, technical and intellectual distance between the Reformers and those who have to implement commissioning and provide the new service ... One is left with the feeling that a key purpose of commissioning is to constrain the existing demand for health-care services (Opit 1993, p. 89).

If patients are to genuinely believe that purchasing authorities are acting in their best interests, it is not enough that purchasers have access to reliable information. Patients must also be able to place their trust in the motivation of purchasing authorities. If the claim of 'money following patients' is not to become a façade for a reality of 'patients following money', the purchasing authorities must reconcile the twin pressures of resource constraints from above with the demands for beneficial patient care from below. To do so successfully requires them to avoid becoming clandestine double agents, nominally acting on behalf of patients but increasingly coerced into making more muddled decisions by sustained unresolved financial pressure from their paymasters.

To reconcile these twin pressures requires instead a more open examination of the effectiveness of different healthcare expenditures in producing beneficial health outcomes. This in turn implies an improved meta-analysis of clinical trial data, a greater dissemination of information about the clinical effectiveness (or ineffectiveness) of different treatments, and the creation of a national register of cost-effectiveness studies.

One of the political assessments behind *Working for Patients* appears to have been that unless there is enforced change, there will be no change. The White Paper rejected a carefully designed and independently evaluated five year programme of controlled experiments to test different ways of breaking the old mould in the most beneficial way. Instead, the ringmaster at the centre of the circus (where even John le Carré located his controller) proceeded simply to crack the whip, with all obedient agents expected to jump through their prescribed hoops. The real world, however, has proved more difficult to stage manage, so that what we have witnessed instead in the first five years has been a breathtaking display of ingenious improvisation in response to the numerous central directives. It is a heart-warming testimony to the resilience and commitment of those concerned. However, as Maréchal Bosquet remarked about the Charge of the Light Brigade, 'C'est magnifique, mais ce n'est pas la guerre!'.

Forcing the pace of innovation in areas like the introduction of new computer systems, in order to support the new world order of the internal market, has itself resulted in a poorly designed central management strategy that has risked being both ineffective and an inefficient waste of resources, as the National Audit Office (NAO) (1990) warned at the time. The risk of less-than-magnificent outcomes from such a forced pace of innovation is underlined by the failure of the London Ambulance Service to respond satisfactorily to emergency calls during a 48 hour period in 1992, following the ill-considered introduction of a new computer system. The subsequent public inquiry blamed the failure on a 'misguided' 'high-risk' managerial decision to pursue the 'ambitious' project under 'an impossible timetable' imposed under an 'over-aggressive' management style (*The Independent*, 26 February 1993).

As Williams (1990b, p. 237–8) noted soon after the publication of *Working For Patients*:

> to extract from this unseemly haste some crumbs of comfort for the future, one might observe that it places a great responsibility on the health services research community to engage in the thinking about the medium term (that is, the next five years) which is otherwise likely to go by default. Whether that thinking will, in the event, prove fruitful will, of course, depend on whether shouldering this responsibility enables the health services research community to attract (largely from Government) the resources necessary to do the work which the Government itself should have commissioned in advance.

The subjects that were thought to be of particular interest to economists were concerned with the behaviour of GP fundholders and of NHS Trusts in the new market structure, the optimal structure of contracts, and what will happen to any slack created by competitive pressure. The impression, more than five years on, is that these market structures have turned out to be far more complex than had been envisaged by their creators, and we are still exploring their properties. Contracts are still extremely crude, because the knowledge required to make them less crude is just not there.

Moreover unresolved tensions exist under the new short-term contracts between the pressure for short-term efficiency savings which one year contracts generate and the achievement of longer term efficiency in the investment of scarce resources in health care facilities. As stressed in Mayston (1992), the assumption of *complete markets* that is involved in the standard theorems of economic theory on the efficiency of competitive markets is notably invalid in the case of the new NHS internal market, where no futures market for the supply of health care beyond the next 12 months or so exists. In the absence of futures markets, market processes can result in inefficient decisions on capacity and other scarce health care resources over time.

Doubts about the long-term direction of the NHS are reinforced by the lack of clarity as to whether the NHS has a strategic plan for its future development. *The Health of the Nation*'s assessment (Department of Health, 1992) of the health care needs of the country is increasingly looking like another exercise in public relations rather than in genuine strategic planning.

Wandering through le Carré style mists of convoluted uncertainty as to where the system as a whole is heading is hardly an appropriate policy for the health care system of a nation. The application of scientific method requires in contrast a more disciplined approach. The first stage in the process of attempting to improve the condition of even an individual patient is that of a sound diagnosis of the original source of the observed problem based upon an extensive knowledge of the relevant scientific disciplines (such as anatomy, physiology, and bio-chemistry). The second stage is a thorough prognosis of the likely course of events with and without different possible interventions. The third stage is the use of surgery only when necessary and when the surgeon has all due skill and experience.

In the case of the NHS Reforms, we have witnessed major surgery, but without much consultation on the appropriate diagnosis and prognosis, or any extensive testing of alternative forms of treatment, before the decision to undertake major surgery was taken. The observed problems that the NHS Review was originally set up to respond to were financial problems in several parts of the NHS, including politically sensitive marginal constituencies in the Southeast of England. A more scientific diagnosis of the source of these problems, based upon the relevant scientific disciplines of public sector economics and public finance, can attribute these problems in large to two main causes (see Mayston, 1990a). The first is the geographical re-distribution of resources in the NHS away from the Southeast and towards more socially deprived regions further from London. The second is the long-term financial pressure from the *relative price effect* that tends to increase the relative cost of a labour-intensive public service, such as the NHS, as real wages rise with economic growth throughout the economy (see Baumol, 1967).

It is questionable whether the NHS Reforms will help to overcome the relative price effect. The NHS Reforms imply more competition between NHS providers, and an associated reduction in the degree of monopsony power that the NHS can exercise in the labour market. There is then a risk of cost-escalation in the NHS actually increasing, possibly in an unstable way, from the increased competition in the health care labour market that the NHS Reforms imply. This is particularly so if the demand for private health care is also increased by any resulting fall in the quality of care on offer from the NHS (see Mayston, 1990a, 1994b).

Similarly, it is questionable whether the NHS Reforms will result in less geographical re-distribution of resources away from the Southeast. The implementation of the NHS Reforms itself requires an explicit resource allocation formula to be applied down to the more detailed local level of individual purchasing health authorities than that involved in the earlier Resource Allocation Working Party (RAWP) allocations to Regional Health Authorities. Such a greater disaggregation to a more local level is itself likely to reveal the need for even more redistribution of resources away from the Southeast (see Carr-Hill *et al.*, 1994), once health care need is explicitly accepted as the guiding principle.

The importance of a careful appraisal of risk in advance of change applies also to many other aspects of the new regime. Thus, while there is now strong financial pressure for the greater use of day cases and keyhole surgery in the NHS, both may involve an increased risk of adverse clinical outcomes without any significant reduction in costs (see Mayston, 1994b), particularly if they are introduced under excessive managerial pressure from above without adequate testing and training. The risk of adverse managerial decisions from the system of capital charging that was introduced by the NHS Review, and the scope for avoiding this risk by a more carefully designed system, are discussed in detail in Mayston (1990b, 1994b). The scope for the introduction of several of the advantages of an internal market within the NHS, whilst avoiding many of its potential disadvantages, are similarly considered in more detail in Mayston (1992).

Health Care Research

An important omission from *Working for Patients* and its associated Working Papers was research. As we have noted earlier, research is important not only in seeking to improve the current state of the world, but also in identifying and avoiding the risks of bad outcomes from ill-considered actions.

The appointment of a new Director of Research and Development (R&D) for the NHS itself occurred two years after the publication of *Working for Patients*, and appears to have been an independent development. The subsequent research strategy has been to devolve a great deal of R&D to the NHS Regions, and to gather up spare residual central resources for a few big targeted enterprises (such as the Cochrane Centre in Oxford, the Centre for Reviews and Dissemination at York, and the Centre for Research in Primary Care at Manchester). There can be grave doubts about the wisdom of fragmenting research responsibilities around the regions, because it is difficult to think of any research topic that is confined in scope to any single region. There may well be some inter-regional variations in the incidence of different conditions, or in cost structures, or in clinical practice, but the causes and consequences of these variations are themselves better investigated from a national rather than a regional perspective. The move towards decentralization here seems to be have been based on the hope that if local people are involved, they are more likely to implement the findings of the research. However, this seems a weak argument, since nationally funded projects can also be spread around geographically if that is thought desirable, without duplicating the overhead costs of running many different commissioning, managing and monitoring operations.

At the same time, the operation of the internal market has led to the re-emergence of an age-old problem, namely the encouragement of *free-riding* when it comes to 'public goods' like R&D. This has long been a problem with industrial training in the private sector, where the inability of firms to enforce indenture type contracts means that they cannot themselves capture the benefits of investing in training for their employees, because they may be poached by other firms, which thereby avoid the training costs. The classic solutions are training levies, public (i.e. tax financed) provision, or charging the trainees directly and letting them bear the risks concerning the future return on their investment. The free-rider problem in NHS R&D has recently been addressed by the Culyer Report in 1994, which noted that individual purchasers of health care in the new NHS are likely to be reluctant to pay higher prices to some suppliers simply to meet the costs of the providers' research activities (which may or may not be of any long-term benefit to them as particular purchasers). The Report therefore recommends that such research be funded 'as a levy on all health care purchasers' allocations and determined annually' (Culyer, 1994, p. 36, para. 3.32). The Report goes on:

> A levy on all health care purchasers will symbolise common ownership of spending plans. In particular it should encourage interest in R&D at the local level and stimulate identification of local priorities. It should also lead to greater interest in and greater understanding of the national R&D agenda and priorities. We have in mind a levy which provides an investment pool to which suitable R&D from any discipline or setting can have access . . . How to do this needs further consideration.

There is a case here for a more wide-ranging reform of the funding of health services research: one which would eliminate both the Medical Research Council (MRC) and the Economic and Social Research Council as players in this field, and create a Health Services Research Council (HSRC) instead, to be funded by the proposed NHS levy proceeds, the existing MRC health services research funds, and by the Department of Health's own research budget. The HSRC should run in both a responsive and a commissioning mode. It should have on its board both experienced researchers from the key disciplines, but also people from the NHS at national and local levels. It would then have the great advantage of being at arm's length both from the Government and from clinical research. It should have responsibility for the training and career structures of researchers as well as for the conduct of research. It should make a point of trying to think five or ten years ahead to identify the problems we shall face when the dust from the current skirmishes has settled.

Conclusion

One must conclude that it still remains a very great pity that the mode by which *Working for Patients* was brought into the world deliberately excluded the health services research community. As a consequence, instead of obtaining a carefully designed 'knowledge-based' set of proposals circulated for widespread comment and further consideration before decisions were reached, what we were sold instead was a 'conviction-based' set of centrally imposed decisions that were imperfectly conceived and inadequately tested in advance of their implementation. 'Act first, think later' is not a motto which should commend itself to any responsible person, particularly when applied to a nation's health care system, and it is hardly the best way to promote beneficial change. We are still grappling with the consequences.

References

AARON, H. (1991) *Serious and Unstable Condition*, Washington DC: Brookings Institute.

ASSOCIATION OF COMMUNITY HEALTH COUNCILS FOR ENGLAND AND WALES (1994) *Fundholding and Access to Hospital Care*, London: ACHC.

AUDIT COMMISSION (1995) *The Doctors' Tale: The Work of Hospital Doctors in England and Wales*, London: HMSO.

BAUMOL, W. (1967) 'Macroeconomics of unbalanced growth', *American Economic Review*, **67**, 3, pp. 415–26.

CARR-HILL, R., HARDMAN, G., MARTIN, S., PEACOCK, S., SHELDON, T. and SMITH, P. (1994) *A Formula For Distributing NHS Revenues Based on Small Area Use of Hospital Beds*, York: Centre for Health Economics, University of York.

CULYER, A.J. (Chairman) (1994) *Supporting Research and Development in the NHS*, London: HMSO.

DEPARTMENT OF HEALTH (1989) *Working For Patients*, Cm 555, London: HMSO.

DEPARTMENT OF HEALTH (1992) *The Health of the Nation*, Cm 1986, London: HMSO.

DEPARTMENT OF HEALTH (1994) *Departmental Report*, Cm 2512, London: HMSO.

KAY, J.A. and THOMPSON, D. (1986) 'Privatisation: a policy in search of a rationale', *Economic Journal*, **96**, 381, pp. 18–32.

KING'S FUND INSTITUTE (1989) *Efficiency in the NHS: A Study of Cost Improvement Programmes*, Occasional Paper No. 2, London: King's Fund Institute.

MAYSTON, D.J. (1990a) 'NHS resourcing: a financial and economic analysis', in CULYER, A.J., MAYNARD, A.K. and POSNETT, J.W. (Eds) *Competition in Health Care*, London: Macmillan.

David Mayston

MAYSTON, D.J. (1990b) 'Managing capital resources in the NHS', in CULYER, A.J.,
    MAYNARD, A.K. and POSNETT, J.W. (Eds) *Competition in Health Care*, London:
    Macmillan.
MAYSTON, D.J. (1992) 'Internal markets, capital and the economics of information',
    Public Money and Management, **12**, 1, pp. 47–53.
MAYSTON, D.J. (1993) 'Principals, agents and the economics of accountability in the new
    public sector', *Accounting, Auditing and Accountability Journal*, **6**, 3, pp. 68–96.
MAYSTON, D.J. (1994a) *Output Indicators in the Public Services*, London: HM Treasury.
MAYSTON, D.J. (1994b) 'Capital and labour markets for health', paper presented to
    Section F (Economics) of the British Association for the Advancement of Science
    Annual Conference, Loughborough, forthcoming in CULYER, A.J. and WAGSTAFF, A.
    (Eds) *Reforming Health Care Systems*, London: Edward Elgar.
NATIONAL AUDIT OFFICE (1990) *Managing Computer Projects in the NHS*, HC22,
    London: HMSO.
NATIONAL AUDIT OFFICE (1992) *Report of the Comptroller and Auditor General on the
    Department of Health Appropriation Accounts*, London: HMSO.
OPIT, L. (1993) 'Commissioning: an appraisal of a new role', in TILLEY, I. (Ed.) *Managing
    the Internal Market*, London: Paul Chapman.
ORGANISATION FOR ECONOMIC COOPERATION AND DEVELOPMENT (1992) *The Reform of
    Health Care: A Comparative Analysis of Seven OECD Countries*, Paris: OECD.
ORGANISATION FOR ECONOMIC COOPERATION AND DEVELOPMENT (1993) *OECD Health
    Systems*, Volumes I and II, Paris: OECD.
ORGANISATION FOR ECONOMIC COOPERATION AND DEVELOPMENT (1994) *The Reform of
    Health Care Systems: A Review of Seventeen OECD Countries*, Paris: OECD.
PACKWOOD, T., KEEN, J. and BUXTON, M. (1991) *Hospitals in Transition*, Milton Keynes:
    Open University Press.
PALMER, A. (1994) 'Carnage in the community', *The Spectator*, 7 May, pp. 9–11.
PUBLIC ACCOUNTS COMMITTEE (1993) *Wessex Regional Health Authority: Management
    of the Regional Information Systems Plan*, Minutes of Evidence, HC 658 i, London:
    HMSO.
ROBINSON, R. and LE GRAND, J. (Eds) (1994) *Evaluating the NHS Reforms*, London:
    King's Fund Institute.
ROTHSCHILD, M. and STIGLITZ, J. (1976) 'Equilibrium in competitive insurance markets:
    an essay in the economics of imperfect information', *Quarterly Journal of
    Economics*, **90**, 4, pp. 629–48.
SENG, C., LESSOF, L. and MCKEE, M. (1993) 'Whose on the Fiddle?', *Health Service
    Journal*, 7 January, pp. 16–17.
WILLIAMS, A. (1990a) 'Ethics, clinical freedom and the doctors' role', in CULYER, A.J.,
    MAYNARD, A.K. and POSNETT, J.W. (Eds) *Competition in Health Care*, London:
    Macmillan.
WILLIAMS, A. (1990b) 'Research implications of the NHS Review', in CULYER, A.J.,
    MAYNARD, A.K. and POSNETT, J.W. (Eds) *Competition in Health Care*, London:
    Macmillan.
YATES, J. (1995) *Serving Two Masters: Consultants, the National Health Service and
    Private Medicine*, London: Channel Four Television.

Chapter 2

Should Alcohol be Taxed for the Public Good?

David Buck, Christine Godfrey and
Gerald Richardson

Introduction

Most countries impose special expenditure taxes on alcohol and there is a long history of high alcohol taxation in the UK. Spirits have attracted a higher rate of tax than other beverages but there is little evidence to suggest that different beverages in themselves have different harmful effects. Along with the historic inconsistencies in tax levels between beverages, it is difficult to discern a clear pattern in the annual budgets that determines any changes in tax levels. Table 2.1 shows the changes to specific alcohol taxes made in the annual UK budget in the past few years. Analysis of budgets suggest that these changes in tax are made for a mixture of immediate revenue needs and possibly in response to industrial lobbying rather than as a means of achieving social policy objectives (Leedham and Godfrey, 1990).

A more recent influence on UK Government taxation policy has been the European Union. Even prior to the creation of a single market and removal of border controls from January 1993, amendments had to be made to UK alcohol tax. The European Commission has argued that beer and wine should be taxed on a similar basis to ensure fair competition for wine, which is mainly imported, compared to beer which is mainly UK produced. In 1984, wine duty was lowered by an amount equivalent to 18p a bottle in order to meet these European requirements. More recently, the abolition of border controls in January 1993 has meant travellers are free to purchase duty paid alcoholic beverages for their personal use in European countries which attract lower rates of tax. The perceived threat of cross border shopping has lead to campaigns by the alcohol industries for a reduction in UK tax rates.

However, the UK Government have also set targets to reduce the numbers

David Buck, Christine Godfrey and Gerald Richardson

drinking inappropriately as part of a major health policy initiative. Taxation policy was seen as a potential instrument that could be used to help achieve these targets. In *The Health of the Nation* policy document (Department of Health, 1992) it is stated that: 'Health will be one of the factors which the Chancellor of the Exchequer will take into account in deciding the appropriate level of alcohol duties in any year.' This is not such a firm statement as has been made in the same policy document for cigarettes, and indeed the current Chancellor (Kenneth Clarke) announced in the 1993 Budget that cigarette duties would be raised by 3 per cent above the rate of inflation for the following three years to achieve better population health.

Despite vigorous lobbying by the trade in 1994, alcohol taxes were not lowered in the November budget. Indeed the taxes were subsequently raised in the mini-budget the Government had to impose to recoup revenue from their defeat on a proposed increase in fuel taxes. These and other past budget decisions suggest that alcohol tax policy is influenced by a number of different economic and political factors. The purpose of this chapter is to examine some of the arguments and evidence for imposing special taxes on alcohol to improve

Table 2.1: Specific duty rates on alcohol 1984–95

Year	Duty per litre of alcohol (£)			
	Beer[1]	Wine[2]	Spirits	Cider[3]
1984	6.96	6.03	15.48	2.38
1985	7.48	6.53	15.77	2.63
1986	7.48	6.53	15.77	2.63
1987	7.48	6.53	15.77	2.63
1988	7.83	6.83	15.77	2.89
1989	7.83	6.83	15.77	2.89
1990	8.44	7.35	17.35	3.11
1991	9.22	8.04	18.96	3.40
1992	9.64	8.40	19.81	3.55
1993	10.11	8.82	19.81	3.73
1993[4]	10.45	–	–	–
1994	10.45	8.98	19.81	3.80
1995[5]	10.82	9.36	20.60	3.96

Source: Adapted from Brewers and Licensed Retailers Association (1994) and Customs and Excise personal communication (1995).

Notes: 1 Assuming average strength to 1993 and 4 per cent abv from then on.
2 Assuming 15 per cent alcohol content.
3 Assuming 6 per cent alcohol content.
4 In June 1993 the method of taxing beer changed, two figures are therefore given for this year.
5 Duty changes which came into effect on 1 January.

society's welfare and how such arguments may influence future policy decisions.

The ability of tax as an intervention to achieve gains in welfare of the population breaks down into a number of different parts. Tax would not be an effective intervention if tax did not affect price, price did not affect consumption and consumption changes were not related to changes in alcohol related problems. The importance of tax as a determinant of the prices of alcohol is considered in the next section along with the evidence of the effect of prices on alcohol consumption. The third section contains a brief review of the complex link between consumption patterns and the health and social effects of inappropriate drinking. In the fourth section the possible costs and benefits arising from taxing alcohol are outlined to give the basis for exploring whether changes in taxes can be judged to be for the public good. In the fifth section the different influences on policy makers and the potential conflict between trade and welfare objectives are explored.

Alcohol Tax, Prices and Consumption

The relationship between alcohol taxes and prices

Alcoholic drinks are subject to two forms of expenditure taxation. Like most consumer goods they are subject to Value Added Tax (VAT) currently set at the rate of 17.5 per cent. This taxation is applied on the final selling price and collected at the retail level. However, all alcoholic drinks also have a specific tax imposed upon them although the nature of these taxes varies across beverages. The specific taxes are levied and collected at the manufacturing and wholesale stage. Any increase in the specific tax, unless absorbed by the manufacturer, will increase the final selling price and hence the amount of VAT paid on each purchase. The specific taxes are set in terms of pence per litre of alcohol and without changes in the annual budget they will lose value. Other things being equal, alcohol prices would in these circumstances fall relative to other goods.

The form of specific taxation varies across beverages. For cider there is a flat rate of tax whether the cider is of low or high alcohol content. For wine there are different tax bands according to strength and type of wine but the rates are constant within the band. Specific taxes on beer and spirits vary directly with alcohol strength. Given this complex structure and historic variations in the level of taxes between beverages, it is not surprising that current levels of tax converted to terms of pure alcohol content rates vary considerably. For average strengths of all beverages, the current specific tax rate converts to £20.60 for spirits, £10.82 for beer, £12.21 for wine and £3.96 for cider for each litre of pure alcohol. Thus, the rate of tax on spirits is nearly twice that of beer and five times that of cider when measured in terms of alcohol content.

David Buck, Christine Godfrey and Gerald Richardson

Specific tax however, is, only one component of price. Different beverages have different costs of manufacture, distributing and retailing costs, and associated profits. Differences in these other components will also affect the final selling price and hence the amount of VAT which will be added at the retail stage. Some of the disparities in specific duty levels are not reflected as large differences in final retail prices but the total tax levied still varies across beverages. Specific taxes and VAT account for approximately 29 per cent of a pint of cider, 32 per cent of the price of a pint of beer, 50 per cent of the price of a bottle of wine and 65 per cent of a bottle of spirits (HM Customs and Excise, 1994).

The impact of tax and therefore tax changes on price levels will vary across the beverages. Also changes in other components of prices will affect final retail prices. In particular, in recent years beer prices have risen much faster than either tax changes or general inflation would have dictated (Richardson and Godfrey, 1993). The trend of changes in tax levels and other components of real prices indicate that specific duty levels for beer remained virtually constant between 1982 and 1993. The real increases in beer prices have been driven by increases in the costs and profits component. For beer, the cost and profit element of price has risen in real terms (at 1990 prices) from approximately 50 pence per pint in 1982 to approximately 80 pence per pint in 1993. As these costs increased, so did the amount of VAT due on each item purchased. For spirits the duty levels have fallen in real terms over the period but this fall has been almost equally compensated by an increase in the costs and profit component. For wine there were small falls in the real duty levels but a more substantial fall in the cost and profit component. For cider, VAT became a more important component of price than the specific tax rate by the end of the period.

This cursory analysis of alcohol prices indicate that tax is a potential means of affecting prices but these prices will also be affected by other factors. The Government's ability to influence prices through taxation is therefore limited.

The relationship between alcohol prices and consumption

Just as taxes are one influence on the level of prices, prices are one factor that determines the overall level of alcohol consumption. Economists generally measure the responsiveness of consumption to price or other changes in terms of elasticities, a price elasticity of -1.0, for example, would suggest that if prices rose by 10 per cent then consumption would fall by 10 per cent, all other factors influencing consumption remaining the same.

There have been many studies of the determinants of alcohol consumption. The majority of studies have used data aggregated across populations and used multiple regression techniques to determine the individual contributions of various factors to changes in alcohol consumption. Price has been found to be an important determinant of the total consumption of alcohol in many countries

(Edwards *et al.*, 1994). Research also suggests that price elasticity estimates vary across beverages and may change over time.

In the UK, the consumption of beer, the UK's favourite drink, used to have the lowest price elasticity, estimated at one point at –0.2 but rapidly rising prices seem to have pushed the estimates upwards in recent years (Godfrey, 1994). The current Treasury estimate for beer price elasticity is –1.0. In contrast, the estimates for price elasticities for spirits and wine, at one time considered luxury items, have fallen. Current Treasury estimates are –1.1 for wine, cider and perry and –0.9 for spirits.

It may be thought that differences in price between beverages would affect their relative popularity. For example, if wine became relatively more expensive than beer or spirits it may be expected that not only would the consumption of wine fall but that more beer and spirits would be drunk. However, estimates suggest that these cross price effects are very small (Godfrey, 1989).

Another concern is whether all groups of drinkers respond in the same way to price changes. It may be suggested, for example, that tax changes and price increases would not affect the heaviest drinkers, possibly because they are dependent on, or addicted to, alcohol. Research, although limited, does not support this hypothesis. For example, research using data from the General Household Survey suggests that there is increasing responsiveness to price the higher the levels of drinking among men aged between 16 and 35 (Sutton and Godfrey, 1994; Sutton and Godfrey, 1995).

Price is one, but not the only, determinant of consumption. Other factors found to influence the overall level of consumption include advertising and availability controls (Edwards *et al.*, 1994). Another important influence is income, and income elasticities for alcohol have been found to be quite high. Thus when incomes are rising, it is likely that taxation policy alone may not be sufficient to stabilize or reduce alcohol consumption levels.

Alcohol, Problems, Individuals and Society

Drinking alcohol is a pleasurable activity for the majority of the population. However, there are also a range of health, social and legal problems associated with alcohol consumption. Some consequences of drinking impact only on the individual drinker (private costs), while others, for example drink-driving or public order disturbances, can impact on other members of society. In economic terms, the impact on third parties are known as external costs or externalities. These private and external costs are not exclusive to the heavy drinker. Drinking in an inappropriate manner, particularly consuming large amounts in single episodes, could result, for example, in an accident, poor performance at work, unsafe sex or violence. For the remainder of the drinking population, there may be few problems and considerable benefits.

David Buck, Christine Godfrey and Gerald Richardson

Mortality

Some of these complex issues can be illustrated by examining the relationship between drinking and health. Chronic drinking is associated with liver problems and some cancers as well as psychological disorders. The number of premature deaths associated with named alcohol disorders is, however, relatively small at about 2000 per year. Alcohol is associated with a much larger range of diseases but is generally one of a number of risk factors. Estimates of the total number of alcohol related deaths per year, using different epidemiological surveys, varies from 9500 to 33000 based on 1991 England and Wales mortality figures (Godfrey and Hardman 1994). These figures translate into between 220000 and 500000 life years lost per year.

Morbidity

As well as premature death, alcohol is a contributory factor to ill-health. This has an impact on the health service with surveys suggesting that a substantial proportion, possibly as many as one in five, of those in hospital may have an alcohol related illness (Barrison *et al.*, 1982; Lockhart *et al.*, 1986). These illnesses also impact on primary care and Accident and Emergency departments, and may result in costs to the NHS of £400 million per year (Godfrey and Maynard, 1992).

Along with the evidence of the harmful effects on health, there is accumulating evidence that moderate drinking, compared to abstinence, may reduce risks from coronary heart disease for middle-aged men and post menopausal women (Marmot and Brunner, 1991; Anderson *et al.*, 1993). This may suggest that there could be some trade-off between the health of some individuals and others in the pursuit of *Health of the Nation* initiatives to reduce alcohol consumption. This evidence has prompted the Government to review its sensible drinking targets but most commentators have suggested that any 'beneficial' effects can be achieved below these limits and as yet the evidence is not strong enough to advise middle-aged male and post menopausal women non drinkers to drink one or two drinks per day (Addiction Research Foundation, 1993; Pearson, 1994).

Estimating the impact of changes in consumption on ill-health is difficult because of the difficulty in finding adequate epidemiological studies that isolate the effect of alcohol on particular diseases. Using the relative risk factors from an Australian review of the international literature, Godfrey and Hardman (1994) attempted to examine the potential impact of inpatient costs in achieving a reduction of consumption levels. The Australian review allowed for an increased risk from heart disease from very low or non-drinkers. Even taking the potential increase in heart disease into account, simulations suggested that there would be gains in life years and savings in alcohol related health service costs if alcohol consumption was reduced. Achieving *Health of the Nation* targets may result in an annual saving of between 30000 and 50000 life years and between £8 million and £11 million in the costs of inpatient care (Godfrey and Hardman, 1994). While health problems largely affect the individual drinker, any excessive health service costs for drinkers impact on third parties in the UK because the National Health Service is publicly funded.

Social costs

Another area which constitutes a major part for estimates of the social costs of alcohol is the impact in the workplace. These costs, like health care costs, can be made up from both individual drinker and external costs. Individual drinkers may lose earnings and risk unemployment, if alcohol affects their productivity or causes sickness absence. Workmates, employers or the taxpayer, however, may also bear some of these costs. The costs can be spread over a wide range of drinking patterns. In a Government drinking survey, all employees were asked if drinking had resulted in any time off work because of a hangover or working below par while at work (Goddard, 1991). Heavier drinkers were more likely to admit to such effects than low or moderate drinkers, but there are far more people in the lower drinking categories. Using a number of assumptions, Godfrey and Hardman (1994) suggest that these self-reported workplace effects alone may result in annual costs between £64 million and £717 million. These may be low estimates because of the stigma attached to admitting such effects. Excess sickness absence among heavy drinkers is likely to add over £1000 million to these totals (Maynard, 1993).

Inappropriate alcohol use has been linked to a range of social problems including partner and child abuse (Edwards *et al.*, 1994). Inappropriate drinking is also linked to a range of offences, and there are links between alcohol consumption and a range of legal problems (Ensor and Godfrey, 1993). These social and legal problems seem to occur across a range of drinking levels although risks tend to increase with drinking levels.

To summarize, alcohol consumption is associated with a range of problems that affect the individual drinking, their families and impact on the rest of society. The relationship between levels of drinking and risk of problems may vary considerably. For some problems the risks may be linear and increase in a straightforward way as drinking increases, for others there may be a threshold effect and problems only occur after some level of drinking. For health problems, J and U-shaped risk curves have been postulated, with non-drinkers and heavier drinkers seemingly at an increased risk compared to low and moderate drinkers. At a population level, however, a recent international review of evidence concluded that overall reductions in alcohol consumption are likely to translate into significant reductions in alcohol related problems (Edwards *et al.*, 1994).

David Buck, Christine Godfrey and Gerald Richardson

Costs and Benefits of Tax Policy

Analysis in the previous section suggested that tax could have some impact on price; price is one factor influencing levels of consumption and that changes in consumption impact on the total levels of alcohol related problems. Tax changes, therefore, may be a means of reducing alcohol related problems in a population. The impact on overall social welfare however requires some analysis of the potential costs of the policy itself, particularly on those individual drinkers who may not cause any alcohol problems. It is also important to consider any equity or fairness issues that may arise from imposing special taxes on alcohol.

Taxation is a recognized policy option where there are external or third party costs to any consumption activity. In an ideal world, those creating external costs would pay the extra taxes and this may result in lower consumption and hence lower social costs; any extra revenue could be used to compensate those third parties suffering the costs. The purpose of these externality based taxes would not be to reduce external costs to zero, rather to reduce them to an 'efficient' level (in economic terms, where the marginal benefit to the individual causing the problems is exactly equal to the sum of the marginal costs imposed on the remainder of society). However, this type of policy would be extremely difficult to impose in practice for alcohol related problems. First, this would require identifying those who caused the problems to third parties. Second, the wide range of these alcohol problems would need to be valued. Both of these steps are impractical.

An alcohol taxation policy based solely on third party costs would ignore the impact of alcohol on the individual. With normal goods it is assumed that consumption decisions take account of the costs of consuming to the individual and therefore the individual harmful effects are not relevant. However, this rests on the assumption that consumers are in a position to best judge their own welfare. It could be argued that some alcohol consumers are not fully aware of the harmful effects and therefore are not fully taking into account the costs of consuming. Tax is one way to 'correct' the information gap.

A more complex problem is dealing with addiction or dependence on alcohol. One definition of addiction is that addicted individuals gain little benefit from drinking. In these circumstances a change in consumption patterns, brought about by tax changes, would produce additional benefits to those addicted by reducing alcohol related problems (Pogue and Sgontz, 1989). More realistic rational addiction models can be used to suggest that tax policies could be welcomed by 'addicts' (Crain *et al.*, 1977).

However, alcohol taxation cannot be restricted to the individuals who are either ill-informed, dependent or causing harm to third parties. Hence, the majority of drinkers who are not in any of these categories will lose some benefits from consuming if taxes are increased. However, for some individuals, such as non-drinkers, there will be an unambiguous increase in welfare as external costs fall. The direction of welfare changes across other groups are less certain, in particular for those drinkers who have few problems. Another 'fairness' issue is whether tax imposes too great a burden on low income families. Alcohol consumption is highly responsive to income changes and, in general, higher income families drink more and pay more tax than low income families. However, some families, whose members both drink heavily and smoke may bear a disproportionate tax burden (Godfrey and Powell, 1990).

A number of non-UK studies have attempted to address these issues of alcohol taxation, and estimate whether specific tax levels are sufficiently high to cover the external costs of inappropriate drinking once some account has been taken of the private costs and benefits of drinking. Richardson and Crawley (1994), for example, compared the social costs of alcohol related problems in Australia to a measure of the benefits of alcohol consumption. Their measure of benefits was based on consumers' willingness to pay for alcohol as a normal good. The results suggested that costs exceeded benefits and hence the tax rate may be too low. This calculation was before any allowance for lack of information or dependence on alcohol among consumers was taken into account. In the UK, however, there are much higher levels of taxation and the results of any full cost-benefit exercise is likely to be more dependent on the assumptions made about consumers' knowledge and behaviour (Godfrey and Maynard 1995).

Tax policies will have other economic consequences. Patterns of employment, trade and Government revenue could also change with different tax policies. There are debates as to whether these economic factors form part of the cost-benefit equation, but from a political perspective, these factors may be the driving force behind tax changes.

Future Tax Policy – Conflict between Social Welfare and Trade Objectives?

The economic model based on social welfare would suggest that an analysis of individual health and social problems, borne not by choice but due to a lack of information or dependence, and wider external costs, should be the basis for the taxation of alcohol. However, partly due to problems of measurement, policy seems to be driven not by these factors, but by the effect that taxation would have on variables such as employment, trade and tax revenue. Recent lobbying in the UK and Europe appears to be directed at these macro-economic factors rather than the effect of alcohol misuse on social welfare. A prime example of this is the cross-border shopping debate, which has arisen since the implementation of the Single European Market (SEM).

Alcohol trade is important to the European Union (EU) with southern states being major wine producers and the northern states having major interests in both beer and spirits production. There are clear national trade interests which affect European taxation policy. Early EU involvement in national tax policy was concerned only with ensuring fair competition for all alcohol industries within Europe requiring EU member states, including the UK, to make some changes to tax structures and rates. It was, however, the move to create the SEM that led to more intensive discussions with the aim of harmonizing duties across Europe. Initially it was argued that a single market for alcohol would only work if tax rates were equal across the whole community. However, the existence of exceptionally large disparities in alcohol taxes across Europe made this unfeasible in the short run. Instead, minimum taxation rates have now been agreed for each type of drink, allowing some states such as the UK to levy rates above the minimum allowable. Health problems related to alcohol have been mentioned as one of the reasons for not lowering tax rates in countries such as the UK, Denmark and Ireland.

With the creation of the SEM from 1 January 1993, travellers across Europe were free to buy duty paid goods for their own personal consumption in any European state and bring them back to their own country. Non-harmonized tax rates create an incentive for the importation of alcohol from countries with lower tax rates to those with higher rates. Indicative limits for such personal consumption were set to help staunch the flow of alcohol and detect those who may be importing goods illegally for resale. However, it is still not clear that such limits can be legally enforced and their levels are difficult to understand. For example, personal consumption for beer is set at 110 litres while only 800 cigarettes are allowed.

Cross-border shopping obviously has implications for alcohol industries in the UK. During 1994 they mounted a significant campaign to lobby for reductions in UK alcohol tax levels to bring them more into line with our European neighbours. This lobbying was unsuccessful in 1994 but the campaign is continuing during 1995. Within Europe the minimum duty levies are being reviewed during 1995. The Maastricht Treaty did give health policy more prominence but the wine lobby is still powerful and it seems unlikely that the minimum tax rates will be substantially raised. The UK Government will therefore have to continue to balance health and trade interests in setting alcohol taxes in the immediate future. These decisions are likely to be substantially influenced by estimates of the size of legal cross-border shopping, illegal smuggling and resale, and the impact of this trade on UK economic interests.

The arguments about the effects of cross-border shopping on the UK alcohol industries are not as straightforward as some sections of the industry claim, however (Buck et al., 1994; Whitbread PLC, 1994). If consumers substitute overseas purchased alcohol for UK-purchased goods, domestic sales, profits and employment will fall. However, there could be different effects between production and retailing industries. Retailing is likely to suffer most, especially in the Southeast. The Brewers and Licensed Retailers' Association (BLRA) are particularly concerned for small off-licenses. However, even within the retailing market, the alcohol market is very segmented and whether the public house, or supermarket trade will suffer a large impact is hard to tell. In contrast to the retailers, alcohol manufacturing industries will only be affected by cross-border shopping if goods purchased overseas are not of UK origin. If UK consumers are simply importing UK brands as pure substitutes there will be no effect on production sales or employment. It is even possible that the production industries may benefit from cross-border shopping if consumers are not merely substituting but increasing their overall consumption of UK-produced products because of the income effect. The UK travel industry will also, unambiguously, benefit from cross-border shopping, in terms of increased employment and profits. The Government however, could, incur substantial costs from cross-border shopping through lost tax revenue and increased enforcement costs.

The true impact of cross-border shopping depends, crucially, on the incentives for both legal and illegal activity. The incentives to engage in cross-border shopping may be very different for various groups of the population. For example, the incentive for those who consume alcohol in public houses may be less than for those who drink solely at home, since the social aspects of drinking are more highly valued. The incentives will depend on price differences and as suggested early in this chapter the tax differences are only one factor in determining final prices. In a comparison of popular brands of alcoholic drink, Buck *et al.* (1994) found that the large differences were for those brands that are marketed as cheaper brands in Europe but as luxury, high price brands in the UK. Potential savings from legal cross-border shopping trips will vary enormously depending on travelling costs and the type of alcoholic goods purchased, and estimated savings could be significantly reduced by these other costs.

A Treasury Committee report on the impact of legal cross-border shopping and potential increases in smuggling suggested that there were some causes for concern, but that the trade was not sufficiently large to alter current taxation levels in the UK (Treasury and Civil Service Committee, 1994). These recommendations seemed to be borne out by the Chancellor's budget decisions at the end of 1994. However, it is clear that social welfare criteria for optimal alcohol taxation levels could conflict with narrower and well articulated trade and industry objectives. Even if it could be demonstrated that there would be major health and social benefits from an increase in alcohol taxation, such a social welfare policy would not be adopted unless there was also a significant increase in taxation levels across Europe.

Conclusion

In this chapter some of the complexities of tracing the effects of alcohol taxation policy on social welfare have been explored. Tax is not the only determinant of prices, and price is only one of the factors influencing alcohol consumption. The links between changes in levels and patterns of consumption, and various health and social problems are still strongly debated and good quality quantitative estimates of effects are hard to find. From an economic perspective there is also a need to consider how far individual costs, as compared to those borne by third parties, are important. Taxation policy itself can bring costs especially to those drinkers not currently causing any problems. While increases in alcohol taxation can be shown to be in the overall public good for a number of countries, no full cost benefit study of the impact of changes in alcohol taxation has been undertaken with UK data. Without further evidence that alcohol taxes would significantly increase individual welfare and reduce third party harm, other considerations are likely to take priority in policy making both in the UK and Europe as a whole.

References

ADDICTION RESEARCH FOUNDATION (1993) *Moderate Drinking and Health*, a joint policy statement based on the International Symposium on Moderate Drinking and Health, Toronto: Addiction Research Foundation of Ontario, Canadian Centre on Substance Abuse.

ANDERSON, P., CREMONA, A., PATON, A., TURNER, C. and WALLACE, P. (1993) 'The risks of alcohol', *Addiction*, **88**, pp. 1493–1508.

BARRISON, I.G., VIOLA, L., MUMFORD, J., MURRAY, R.M., GORDON, M. and MURRAY-LYON, I.M. (1982) 'Detecting excessive drinking among admissions to a general hospital', *Health Trends*, **14**, pp. 80–3.

BREWERS AND LICENSED RETAILERS ASSOCIATION (BLRA) (1994) *Statistical Handbook 1994: A compilation of drinks industry statistics*, London: BLRA.

BUCK, D., GODFREY, C. and RICHARDSON, G. (1994) *Should cross-border shopping affect tax policy?*, YARTIC Occasional Paper 6, York: Centre for Health Economics and Leeds Addiction Unit, University of York.

CRAIN, M., DEATON, T., HOLCOMBE, R. and TOLLISON, R. (1977) 'Rational choice and the taxation of sin', *Journal of Public Economics*, **8**, pp. 239–45.

DEPARTMENT OF HEALTH (1992) *The Health of the Nation*, Cm 1986, London: HMSO

EDWARDS, G., ANDERSON, P., BABOR, T.F., CASSWELL, S., FERRENCE, R., GIESBRECHT, N., GODFREY, C., HOLDER, H., LEMMENS, P., MAKELA, K., MIDANIK, L., NORSTROM, T., OSTERBERG, E., ROMELSJO, A., ROOM, R., SIMPURA, J. and SKOK, O-J. (1994) *Alcohol policy and the public good*, Oxford: Oxford University Press.

ENSOR, T. and GODFREY, C. (1993) 'Modelling the interactions between alcohol, crime and the criminal justice system', *Addiction*, **88**(4), pp. 477–487.

GODDARD, E. (1991) *Drinking in England and Wales in the late 1980's*, London: HMSO.

GODFREY, C. (1989) 'Factors influencing the consumption of alcohol and tobacco', *British Journal of Addiction*, **84**, pp. 1123–1138.

GODFREY, C. (1994) 'Economic influences on change on population and personal substance behaviour', in EDWARDS, G. and LADER, M. (Eds) *Addiction: Processes of*

Change, Oxford Medical Publications, pp. 163–187, Oxford.

GODFREY, C. and HARDMAN, G. (1994) *Changing the Social Costs of Alcohol: Final Report to the AERC*, York: Centre for Health Economics.

GODFREY, C. and MAYNARD, A. (1992) *A health strategy for alcohol: setting targets and choosing policies*, YARTIC Occasional Paper 1, York: Centre for Health Economics and Leeds Addiction Unit, University of York.

GODFREY, C. and MAYNARD, A. (1995) 'Economic Evaluation of alcohol policies', in EDWARDS, G. and HOLDER, H. (Eds) *The Scientific Rationale for Alcohol Policy*, Oxford: Oxford University Press.

GODFREY, C. and POWELL, M. (1990) 'The relationship between individual choice and Government policy in the decision to consume hazardous goods', in BALDWIN, S., GODFREY, C. and PROPPER, C. (Eds) *Quality of Life: Perspectives and Policies*, pp. 201–217, London: Routledge.

HM CUSTOMS AND EXCISE (1994) *HM Customs and Excise Annual Report 1993–94*, London: HMSO.

LEEDHAM, W. and GODFREY, C. (1990) 'Tax policy and budget decisions', in MAYNARD, A. and TETHER, P. (Eds) *Preventing Alcohol and Tobacco Problems. Volume 1. The Addiction Market: Consumption, Production and Policy Development*, Aldershot: Avebury/Gower, pp. 96–116.

LOCKHART, S.P., CARTER, Y.H., STRAFFEN, A.M., PANG, K.K., McLOUGHLIN, J. and BARON, J.H. (1986) 'Detecting alcohol consumption as a cause of emergency general medical admissions', *Journal of the Royal Society of Medicine*, **79**(3), pp. 132–6.

MARMOT, M. and BRUNNER, E. (1991) 'Alcohol and cardiovascular disease: the status of the U shaped curve', *British Medical Journal*, **303**, pp. 565–8.

MAYNARD, A. (1993) *Is it helpful to measure the social costs of alcohol use?* YARTIC newsletter 2, York: Centre for Health Economics, University of York and Leeds Addiction Unit.

PEARSON, T.A. (1994) 'What to advise patients about drinking alcohol', *Journal of the American Medical Association*, **272**(12), pp. 967–8.

POGUE, T.F. and SGONTZ L.G. (1989) 'Taxing to control social costs: The case of alcohol', *American Economic Review*, **79**(1), pp. 235–43.

RICHARDSON, J. and CRAWLEY, S. (1994) 'Optimum alcohol taxation: balancing consumption and external costs, *Health Economics*, **3**, pp. 73–87.

RICHARDSON, G. and GODFREY, C. (1993) *Taxing for Health*, Budget submission prepared for Alcohol Concern, York: Centre for Health Economics.

SUTTON, M. and GODFREY, C. (1994) *The Health of the Nation Targets for Alcohol: A Study of the Economic and Social Determinants of High Alcohol Consumption in Different Population Groups*. Report to the Health Education Authority, York: Centre for Health Economics, University of York and Leeds Addiction Unit.

SUTTON, M. and GODFREY, C. (1995) 'A grouped data regression approach to estimating economic and social influences on individual drinking behaviour', *Health Economics*, **4**(3), pp. 237–47.

TREASURY AND CIVIL SERVICE COMMITTEE (1994) *First Report: Cross Border Shopping* vols I–II, London: HMSO.

WHITBREAD PLC (1994) *Cross-channel shopping: The facts*, London: Whitbread PLC.

Chapter 3

The Changing Response to Homelessness

Peter McLaverty, David Rhodes and Hilary Third

Introduction

In January 1994, the Government published the Green Paper *Access to Local Authority and Housing Association Tenancies: A Consultation Paper* (Department of the Environment, 1994a). The document proposed changes to the way in which local authorities should discharge some of their housing duties. Whilst the consultation paper contained wide-ranging recommendations, the specific aim of this chapter is to consider the proposal for local authorities to accommodate homeless households in the private rented sector. Drawing on several pieces of research recently completed in the Centre for Housing Policy, at the University of York, three crucial issues that arise from this proposal will be considered. Firstly, access to the private rented sector for homeless households; secondly, meeting rent payments in the private sector; and thirdly, the future of the private rented sector.

The first part of this chapter discusses the context of the new proposals. This section includes a description of the existing legal framework for housing the statutorily homeless and the main elements of the consultation paper, including reasons why the changes have been proposed. The feasibility of the proposal to increase the use of the private rented sector is evaluated in the light of recent research evidence in the second part of this chapter, and includes landlords' letting preferences, and paying rent in the private rented sector. The third part of this chapter discusses possible future prospects for the private rented sector as a whole. The final part of the paper sets out the main conclusions.

Context

The Housing Act 1985 (Part III) currently requires local authorities to provide permanent accommodation for statutorily homeless households in either council housing or housing association accommodation. To be accepted as statutorily homeless by a local authority, households must fulfill the following four criteria: a household must be homeless or threatened with homelessness within 28 days; it must be in priority need (defined as families with dependent children, pregnant women, and people who are vulnerable due to age or mental or physical illness); the household must not be intentionally homeless; and there must be a local connection. For households with an immediate accommodation need, a local authority will generally provide temporary accommodation (in hostels or bed and breakfast establishments, for example), whilst the application is investigated to ascertain if the household fulfils the criteria to be accepted as statutorily homeless.

Since the introduction of the Housing (Homeless Persons) Act 1977, annual acceptances of homeless households by local authorities have more than doubled, from 60400 in 1980 to 124600 in 1994. Households accepted as statutorily homeless are given priority over other households applying for social housing. Research shows that, on average, homeless households are accommodated about twice as quickly as other applicants, and that approaching half of new social housing lettings are allocated to the homeless (Prescott-Clarke *et al.*, 1994). This increase in local authority acceptances has led to a growing proportion of the total social housing stock being allocated to the homeless, from 20 per cent of all lettings in 1986, to 29 per cent in 1991 (ibid.). In particular, the proportion of the social housing stock allocated to homeless households in London is especially high.

Local authorities usually allow households on their general waiting list the option of refusing up to two reasonable offers of accommodation: that is, non-homeless applicants can often have a choice of three properties before they incur some penalty (Bines *et al.*, 1993). The survey of social housing management, by Bines *et al.*, also found that homeless applicants did not usually have this choice. The code of guidance for homelessness legislation states that: 'A single offer of suitable accommodation normally discharges an authority's responsibilities' (Department of the Environment, 1991). Therefore, whilst the homeless are given priority for permanent housing, they are not usually offered a choice of accommodation.

The new proposals are based on the fundamental premise that the existing allocation of social rented housing is unfair. The consultation paper states that:

> Ministers see no good reason why a person accepted as statutorily homeless should have priority in the allocation of what is in effect

housing for life over people who remain in unsatisfactory accommodation until their turns come up on a waiting list. (Department of the Environment, 1991: Para 2.8)

The proposals contained in the consultation paper attempt to redress the imbalance in the current requirement for local authorities to give a 'fast track' priority to homeless households. A single general waiting list is proposed for all applicants, to be: '... the sole route by which people may be allocated a secure local authority tenancy or may be nominated by a local authority for a similar housing association tenancy' (Department of the Environment, 1994a). Furthermore, the new proposals are based on the belief that being homeless should not of itself be a sufficient condition for a household to be given priority for a permanent tenancy in social rented accommodation. A Department of the Environment (DoE) *News Release* (1994b) states that the intention is to:

ensure that there is a proper safety net for families and vulnerable people who are homeless by creating a new duty on local authorities to provide accommodation for at least a year, during which time their needs would be considered on the same basis as others on the waiting list.

Thus, there will continue to be a safety net function provided by local authorities for households in emergency situations, but this need only be in temporary rather than permanent accommodation. This change will sever the link between statutory homelessness and automatic priority for permanent social housing.

Coupled to these basic aims of the new proposals, the consultation paper makes clear the intention to require local authorities to discharge their housing duties: '... through increasing provision in the private rented sector'. In the DoE *News Release* (1994b), details of the proposal to increase the use of the private rented sector for homeless households were expanded. Local authorities are to be encouraged to develop partnerships with the private rented sector, and there is to be an emphasis on developing rent guarantee (or rent deposit) schemes to help households gain entry to private lettings.

There were an unprecedented 10000 responses to the consultation paper, most of which were in opposition to the proposals. As a result, some of the recommendations in the consultation paper were amended in the DoE *News Release*. For example, the proposed duty on local authorities to provide temporary accommodation for a minimum period of six months was increased to one year. However, the emphasis on using the private rented sector to house homeless households has remained.

Many of the responses to the new proposals expressed concern about using the private rented sector to house homeless families. The attention of these responses was often focused on issues such as standards of accommodation and tenure insecurity in the private sector. Clearly these are important concerns, but very little attention has been given to how feasible it might be to use the private rented sector at all. Therefore, the aim of this paper is to cor housing homeless households in the private rented sector, b findings of some recent research. Before looking at the l however, a brief overview of the private rented sector is set c to contextualize the discussion.

The Private Rented Sector

Boviard *et al.* (1985) and others (for example, Kemp, 1988), have argued that the private rented sector is currently an important tenure for four key demand groups: the first, a slowly declining group of largely elderly people who have always lived in the sector; the second, the young and mobile, for whom the private sector provides flexibility and relative ease of access; the third, employment linked accommodation; and the fourth, the sector performs a residual role, accommodating low income households who have difficulty gaining access to social rented housing or owner occupation. In particular, the new proposals for housing the homeless will utilize this latter function of the private rented sector.

At the beginning of this century, the private rented sector formed the majority tenure, when nine out of every ten households rented from private landlords. However, the sector has continuously declined, and now accommodates about one in ten of all households. During the 1980s, Government attention turned to ways in which the private rented sector could be revitalized, and as a result several measures were introduced in an attempt to stimulate the supply of privately rented dwellings.

A supply-side measure of particular importance was the introduction of the 1988 Housing Act. This Act deregulated all new lettings after 1 January 1989 in England and Wales (and after 15 January 1989 in Scotland), and introduced new-style assured shorthold tenancies. This legislation means that since 1989, deregulation has allowed private landlords to charge market rents, and by using assured shorthold tenancies landlords can be sure of repossession after a minimum let of six months. Further to the 1988 Act, an accelerated possession procedure was introduced on 1 November 1993. This procedure allows landlords to regain possession of their property let on assured shorthold tenancies and, under certain conditions, has assured tenancies much more quickly than before. An additional supply-side measure aimed at stimulating the private rented sector was the extension of the Business Expansion Scheme to companies providing residential lettings on assured tenancies. This scheme, which ran from 1988 to 1993, provided tax incentives to investors in rental housing companies.

Access to the private rented sector

Compared with social rented housing and owner occupation, the private rented sector is often viewed as the tenure of easy access. To live in the private rented sector does not require application to a waiting list, or an assessment of priority need; neither is it necessary to secure a mortgage or employ a solicitor. However, there can still be substantial barriers to gaining entry to a private letting.

The requirement of many landlords for payments of rent in advance and deposits, often totalling several hundred pounds, can present an obstacle to many low income households. This problem is likely to be particularly acute for homeless households, who may not have the substantial financial resources necessary to draw on for rent in advance or deposits. Evidence from research into the bottom end of the private rented sector in Glasgow suggests that schemes to help with advance payments may well be necessary if low income households are to gain access to the private rented sector. The vast majority of tenants living in houses of multiple occupation in Glasgow had paid rent in advance, a deposit, or (most commonly) both; the average payments being £148 for rent in advance and £118 for a deposit (Kemp and Rhodes, 1994a). Thus, there are often substantial financial costs to gaining entry to even the cheapest forms of privately rented accommodation. A recent survey of single homeless people (that is, non-statutorily homeless people) in England found that one of the main difficulties experienced by those interviewed was their inability to pay a deposit or rent in advance (Anderson *et al.*, 1993).

Clearly, these advance costs present a potential barrier to gaining access to the private rented sector for homeless people (most of whom are not in work) particularly since the introduction of the discretionary cash-limited Social Fund in April 1988. This social security change removed the system of single payments for exceptional needs, making it more difficult for low income households to secure help with the advance charges frequently required by private sector landlords. Under the Social Fund it is no longer possible to obtain money for deposits, unlike in the previous system of single payments, but loans or grants may be given for rent in advance. Only 7 per cent of the tenants surveyed in the lower end of Glasgow's private rented sector had applied to the Social Fund for a loan (which was repayable) or a grant, for help with rent in advance. Furthermore, the applications of most of those who had applied to the Social Fund had been refused (Kemp and Rhodes, 1994a). Other large-scale research into the Social Fund also shows that the take-up of loans or grants for rent in advance has been very low (Huby and Dix, 1992). Clearly, however, there is Government awareness of this potential difficulty, as noted in the 1994 DoE *News Release*.

Despite acknowledgement by the Government of the problem of advance payments, and their desire to encourage the development of schemes to help households gain access to private lettings, there is evidence to suggest that homeless households may face other obstacles in securing privately rented accommodation. Research shows that the vast majority of statutorily homeless households are not in paid employment, but are reliant on state benefits of one type or another (Evans and Duncan, 1988). In terms of economic status, these are one of the types of tenant to whom many private landlords are most reluctant to let. A nationally representative survey of private landlords in Scotland (Kemp and Rhodes, 1994b) shows that the landlords of 36 per cent of private sector addresses, which accounted for the largest single response, least preferred to let to unemployed people. Furthermore, almost half the landlords (48 per cent) said their most preferred type of tenants were people in work. These findings are mirrored in research on private landlords in Britain: 29 per cent least preferred to let to unemployed people, and 49 per cent most preferred to let to employed people (Crook *et al.*, 1995). Thus, homeless households are unlikely to be the preferred choice of tenant for many landlords.

There has also been research into private landlords' attitudes towards tenants in receipt of housing benefit. Table 3.1 shows that Scottish landlords clearly preferred not to let to housing benefit tenants (a finding echoed by Crook *et al.*, 1995 in Britain). This finding has major implications for statutory homeless households, as the majority of them are in receipt of housing benefit (Prescott-Clarke *et al.*, 1994).

A variety of reasons were given by the Scottish landlords for their preference for non-housing benefit tenants. Eighteen per cent mentioned problems with the bureaucracy of the housing benefit system, and 17 per cent mentioned the delays in the processing of claims as the reason for their preference. Crook *et al.* (1995) also found that landlords' preferences for non-housing benefit tenants were often related to problems with the administration of the system: landlords in Britain commonly preferred not to let to housing benefit tenants because of the 'red tape' and 'hassles' involved. A qualitative survey of private landlords and restrictions in eligible rents for housing benefit in England and Wales (Bevan *et al.* 1995), also found that landlords and letting agents had commonly experienced

Table 3.1: Landlords' preferences for housing benefit or non-housing benefit tenants

Preference	Total landlords (%)
Prefer housing benefit tenants	4
Prefer non-housing benefit tenants	58
No preference	38
(Base)	(275)

Source: Kemp and Rhodes (1994b)

difficulties because of delays in the processing of claims.

However, the Scottish landlords who preferred not to let to housing benefit tenants most commonly gave reasons which were associated with their perception of housing benefit tenants (Kemp and Rhodes, 1994b). Twenty per cent said that the rent was not always paid or that housing benefit was spent on other things; 20 per cent said that housing benefit tenants do not look after the property; and 18 per cent said that housing benefit tenants were undesirable (more than one response could be given). Clearly, therefore, housing benefit administration is a major source of difficulty for private landlords, and one which may affect their letting preferences. However, even if a requirement of the local authorities lies in ensuring prompt payment of housing benefit to homeless households in the private sector (Department of the Environment, 1994a), evidence suggests that many private landlords may still be unwilling to let to people in receipt of housing benefit because of their views on the tenants themselves.

Paying rent in the private rented sector

Once access has been gained to private sector accommodation, meeting the regular payments of rent is of paramount importance. Rent arrears can cause major financial difficulties for landlords, who may have no option other than to evict tenants who get into serious arrears (Bevan *et al.* 1995). As noted above, the majority of statutorily homeless households are in receipt of housing benefit. However, this situation does not automatically mean that these households will have all their rent covered by housing benefit, and many may have to make a contribution towards their rent from other sources of income.

At the present time, local authority housing benefit sections have to send claims from private sector tenants to the local Rent Officer Service. The rent officer then determines whether the rent is significantly above a reasonable market rent level and whether it is unreasonably large for the claimant's needs. If the rent is deemed over expensive or the accommodation over large, the rent officer has to determine a reasonable market rent for the accommodation, or a notional rent based on a reasonable market rent for the size of accommodation the claimant should occupy. The local authority then has to decide whether to pay the full contractual rent claimed, or to simply pay up to the reasonable market rent level determined by the rent officer.

On payments up to the rent officer determined reasonable market rent level, local authorities receive a subsidy of 95 per cent from the Department of Social Security. However, if local authorities pay above the reasonable market rent determined by the rent officer, they receive no subsidy on the amount above the figure, unless a member of the household is in a protected group (that is, a person aged 60 or over, or a dependent child, or someone unable to work for social security purposes due to sickness or disability) in which case they receive a 60 per cent subsidy.

While local authorities are supposed to make an independent assessment of a claimant's individual position, research shows that for 86 per cent of private sector housing benefit claims, local authorities were using the rent officer determined reasonable market rent as the eligible rent for housing benefit (Kemp and McLaverty, 1994). In the financial year 1992/3, over two-fifths of rents referred to the Rent Officer Service (44 per cent) were determined to be over expensive, or the accommodation over large. In these cases, the average difference between the contractual rent and the reasonable market rent determined by the rent officer was £910 per annum (Department of the Environment, 1993).

If the general housing benefit regulations are applied to the homeless housed in privately rented accommodation, many are likely to find that housing benefit does not meet their full contractual rent. This 'rent gap' may mean that many households will have to make up the difference, or fall into arrears. Taking the average annual 'rent gap' of £910 featured in the previous example, this situation may mean that, after the April 1995 benefits uprating, an unemployed lone parent aged over 18 with one child under the age of 11, would have to find £17.50 (£910/52) per week from a total weekly income of £77.95 (£46.55 personal allowance + £15.95 allowance for a child under 11 + £10.25 family premium + £5.20 lone parent premium). Furthermore, some households may find themselves in serious arrears as a result of delays in the processing of housing benefit claims, as they may not be aware that their housing benefit entitlement does not cover the full contractual rent until the processing of the claim is completed.

A further probable outcome of accommodating more homeless people in the private rented sector would be an increase in the workload of council housing benefit sections. This situation might arise because it is much harder for housing benefit staff to determine housing benefit payments for private sector tenants than for council tenants. Research has shown that 17 per cent of councils in 1992 said they did not meet the statutory time limits for initial payments to private sector claimants, whilst among inner London boroughs the figure was 31 per cent (Kemp and McLaverty, 1994). A 1991 survey found that 20 per cent of councils were not making interim payments even when required by law to do so (Kemp, 1992). Without increased staffing levels, many local authorities would find it very difficult to guarantee payments to landlords of ex-homeless people within a certain time period – unless, that is, payments for other claimants were delayed.

Future Prospects for the Private Rented Sector

Since the 1988 Housing Act, there has been a small reversal in the continual decline of the private rented sector. After reaching an all-time low of 8.6 per cent in 1989, the proportion of privately renting households had increased to 9.4 per cent at the time of the 1991 Census. Evidence shows that the private rented sector has continued to slowly expand since 1991, accounting for 9.9 per cent of all households in 1993 (Downs *et al.*, 1994). However, there has been some debate about the extent to which this small increase can be attributed to the supply-side policy initiatives (the 1988 Housing Act, the extension of Business Expansion Schemes for assured tenancies, and the accelerated possession procedure) or to the slump in the owner occupied housing market. If the expansion in the private rented sector is largely due to the property slump, with many landlords letting as a temporary measure until prices improve, then there may in time be a net reduction in the size of the sector. Clearly, the sustainability, if not the continued expansion, of the private rented sector is of crucial importance if local authorities are to be able to increase their reliance upon it.

There is evidence to suggest that at least some private landlords are reluctant landlords, who may withdraw from letting if the housing market improves. Crook *et al.* (1995) found that 5 per cent of the private individual landlords they interviewed regarded the address of their letting(s) as their home which they were unable or unwilling to sell at present. Similarly, 3 per cent of Scottish landlords regarded their property in the same way (Kemp and Rhodes, 1994b). However, if many reluctant landlords are using letting agencies rather than managing their property themselves, and there is some evidence to suggest that many are (Bevan *et al.*, 1995), the proportion of private landlords who may withdraw from letting if the housing market improves could be much higher. A 1993 survey of letting agents found that almost one fifth of the private individual landlords whose property they were managing (18 per cent), were reluctant landlords (Rhodes, 1993). This proportion of landlords is not an insignificant figure, as almost three fifths of British landlords were private individuals, and only a very small minority of these were full-time landlords (Crook *et al.*, 1995).

If the private sector is to expand as the Government wishes, landlords and potential landlords would probably require rates of return that encouraged them to let accommodation. The Government deregulated private sector rents in the 1988 Act for that reason. However, with fair rents being replaced by market rents for all tenancies started after 1 January 1989, and with economic recession, the housing benefit bill has reached higher levels. As part of its efforts to reduce the public sector borrowing requirement, the Government is currently looking at ways of reducing the amount spent on housing benefit. However, the Government's plans to reduce the public sector borrowing requirement by altering the housing benefit system may come into conflict with the policy initiative to rehouse homeless people in the private rented sector.

The Government is proposing to introduce local 'reference rents' for new housing benefit claims in October 1995. The latest information available indicates that the reference rents will be determined by the rent officer service to reflect local housing markets. All deregulated private sector rents, excluding extreme outliers, will be taken into consideration, with the mid-point in the range of rents to be taken as the local reference rent. Housing benefit entitlement will continue to be assessed as it is now, up to the reference rent level, but for rents above this level, however, housing benefit payments will be restricted to half the difference between the reference rent and the contractual rent. Furthermore, the present rules regarding housing benefit payments to vulnerable claimants are to be discontinued, with local authorities being given discretion to make payments above the rent officer determined rent in cases where the contractual rent is higher than the determination.

The aim of this policy is to encourage claimants to find cheaper accommodation. However, the policy change is unlikely to encourage potential private landlords to put property on the rental market. Even amongst existing landlords in Britain, more than two-fifths said that the rent they were receiving was insufficient (Crook *et al.*, 1995). The average net rate of return thought to be necessary to attract new investment into the private rented sector by the Association of Residential Letting Agents members was 10.4 per cent, a figure that compares with an average achieved net rate of return of 6.7 per cent (Rhodes, 1993). This difference equates to a gap of 3.7 per cent net, which was thought to be necessary to attract new private sector investment. Crook *et al.* (1995) found a similar 'yield gap' in their survey of private landlords.

If landlords feel they have to charge rents at certain levels in order to make what they regard as satisfactory financial returns, and the reference rents on individual housing benefit claims are below those levels, two results are possible: first, the revival of the private rented sector is likely to be adversely affected; and second, claimants may face acute difficulty in affording their rent. The availability of private sector accommodation for homeless people would probably decrease in such a situation, as homeless people are particularly unlikely to have resources, or access to them, to make up any difference between their contractual rent and the housing benefit they receive.

Conclusions

Homeless households are likely to face difficulty in gaining entry to the private rented sector for purely financial reasons. It is clear that schemes to help with paying rent in advance and deposits would, as acknowledged by the Government, perform an important role in enabling low income households to help meet these access costs. However, the homeless are also likely to face another major obstacle, namely, widespread reluctance amongst private landlords to let to people in receipt of housing benefit or those who are unemployed. Housing benefit, in particular, is a source of concern for many private landlords, who not only have negative views of the system itself, but who often prefer not to let to housing benefit tenants because of their perceptions of the tenants themselves.

Meeting rents may also cause difficulties for many homeless households accommodated in the private rented sector, particularly as serious rent arrears can lead to evictions. Where housing benefit does not cover the full contractual rent, low income households could have difficulty meeting the shortfall between their housing benefit entitlement and the total rent. This situation may result in rent arrears, especially in cases where the arrears have built up due to delays in the processing of housing benefit claims. Furthermore, the likely increased workload on housing benefit staff, who find it most difficult to process private sector claims, may exacerbate the problem of delays.

Even though the private rented sector has slightly increased in size in recent years, it is unclear if it has the spare capacity to accommodate more people. What can be said, however, is that there are at least some reluctant private landlords who are likely to withdraw from letting if values improve and transactions increase in the owner occupied housing market. In addition, the implementation of reference rents for housing benefit in October 1995, which depends on the level at which they are set, may conflict with the proposal for local authorities to make increasing use of the private sector. It is clear that many private landlords are not satisfied with the level of rents they can charge and any reduction in rent levels as a result of changes to the housing benefit system, far from encouraging new landlords into the market, may force many existing landlords to exit from the sector.

References

ANDERSON, I., KEMP, P.A. and QUILGARS, D. (1993) *Single Homeless People*, London: HMSO.

BEVAN, M., KEMP, P.A. and RHODES, D. (1995) *Private Landlords and Restrictions in Eligible Rents*, York: Centre for Housing Policy.

BINES, W., KEMP, P.A., PLEACE, N. and RADLEY, C. (1993) *Managing Social Housing*, London: HMSO.

BOVIARD, A., HARVOE, M. and WHITEHEAD, C.M.E. (1985), 'Private rented housing: its current role', *Journal of Social Policy*, **14**, 1, pp. 1–23.

CROOK, A.D.H., HUGHES, J. and KEMP, P.A. (1995) *The Supply of Privately Rented Homes: Today and Tomorrow*, York: Joseph Rowntree Foundation.

DEPARTMENT OF THE ENVIRONMENT (1991) *Homelessness Code of Guidance for Local Authorities*, London: HMSO.

DEPARTMENT OF THE ENVIRONMENT (1993) *English House Condition Survey: 1991*, London: HMSO.

DEPARTMENT OF THE ENVIRONMENT (1994a) *Access to Local Authority and Housing Association Tenancies: A Consultation Paper*, London: DoE.

DEPARTMENT OF THE ENVIRONMENT (1994b) *News Release 421*, July.

DOWNS, D., HOLMANS, A. and SMALL, H. (1994) *Trends in the Size of the Private Rented Sector in England*, London: HMSO.

EVANS, A. and DUNCAN, S. (1988) *Responding to Homelessness: Local Authority Policy and Practice*, London: HMSO.

HOUSING ACT 1988, London: HMSO.

HUBY, M. and DIX, G. (1992), *Evaluating the Social Fund*, London: HMSO.

KEMP, P.A. (1988) *The Future of Private Renting*, Salford: University of Salford.

KEMP, P.A. (1992) *Housing Benefit: An Appraisal*, London: HMSO.

KEMP, P.A. and McLAVERTY, P. (1994) 'The Determination of Eligible Rents for Housing Benefit: the Implementation by Local Authorities of Central Government Policy', *Environment and Planning C: Government and Policy*, No. 12, pp. 109–122.

KEMP, P.A. and RHODES, D. (1994a) *The Lower End of the Private Rented Sector: A Glasgow Case Study*, Edinburgh: Scottish Homes.

KEMP, P.A. and RHODES, D. (1994b) *Private Landlords in Scotland*, Edinburgh: Scottish Homes.

PRESCOTT-CLARKE, P., CLEMENS, S. and PARK, A. (1994) *Routes into Local Authority Housing: A Study of Local Authority Waiting Lists and New Tenancies*, London: HMSO.

RHODES, D. (1993) 'The State of the Private Rented Sector', Joseph Rowntree Housing Research, *Findings*, No. 90.

Chapter 4

Costs and Benefits of Treating Drug Problems

Christine Godfrey and Matthew Sutton

Introduction

The consumption of illicit drugs receives considerable media attention. Interventions by the police and HM Customs and Excise which are directed at interrupting the drugs trade account for the majority of Government resources devoted to tackling drug-related problems (Sutton and Maynard, 1994). Efforts to reduce the demand for illicit drugs through prevention or treatment receive considerably less financial priority, but factors such as the potential spread of the HIV-virus through drug users sharing needles has had a considerable influence on the numbers and types of services available to those seeking help with drug problems.

Some drug treatments are directed at helping a drug user become drug free, and others aim only to minimize the harm associated with drug use. The prescription of substitute drugs is one treatment option that is receiving considerable attention. The most widespread intervention of this type is the prescription of methadone to dependent users of heroin. These types of programmes aim to allow users to regain control over aspects of their lives and reduce the need to illicitly purchase drugs. However, methadone and other substitute drugs are still controlled substances and these programmes remain controversial.

The benefits of drug treatment are largely considered by clinicians in terms of the individual or family involved. For the user, the treatment may improve health, social functioning and lead to greater employment opportunities. However, as acknowledged by both governments and drug treatment agencies, drug treatments can also involve considerable social benefits. For example, this was explicitly noted in a statement of Government drugs policy: '[h]elping drug misusers to give up taking drugs is beneficial both to individuals and for society as a whole' (Home Office, 1990: p. 19). For society, reducing the crime involved in financing drug use is seen as one of the major potential benefits from increased services to drug users. Nevertheless, the financing of drug services requires scarce resources, with the majority of services being financed through the health service. There is a need to ensure that such services are cost-effective. However, different treatment, prevention or enforcement interventions result in a different mix of individual and societal benefits, as well as involving different levels of resources. Moreover, there may be differential gains for some individuals or groups of individuals (such as drug users, victims of drug-related crimes, not-yet-users, and society in general) and losses for others. These issues are particularly pertinent to substitute drug prescribing programmes.

From an economic perspective, the aims of this chapter are to discuss two issues: what is the optimal solution in terms of possible trade-offs between individual and societal benefits and costs? and, if health professionals are to decide on the range of treatment service available, are optimal levels and types of service likely to be provided? To provide some arguments to answer these questions, the costs and benefits of drug use to the individual and to society are considered. In the light of these costs and benefits, the individual drug user has to decide whether to seek help from available services, and society faces choices about what types and volume of services to provide. The individual and societal costs and benefits of one treatment, methadone maintenance therapy, are used in this chapter to illustrate potential trade-offs between different individuals and society in these choices. If trade-offs exist then some 'rules' may be required. Medical and simple economic rules may lead to different conclusions and the impacts of different ethical viewpoints are considered in the final part of the chapter.

Effects of Illicit Drug Use on Individuals and Society

There are many different types of drug user, and some individuals may never pass the stage of experimentation. Gilman and Pearson (1991) describe five *states of involvement* with illicit drugs: non-user; experimentation; occasional use on a recreational basis; 'grey area' of transitional use; and habitual/compulsive/addicted use. At the experimentation stage, it is clear that the consumption of any illicit substance has (perceived) benefits to the individual, be they in terms of mood-alteration, social benefits (such as relief of peer-pressure), or relief of boredom. In an economic rational choice framework, individuals will only consume illicit drugs if the perceived benefits are judged to be greater than the perceived costs. In this paper, dependent users are considered, since these users are traditionally the only group eligible for intensive treatment programmes.

Even for those dependent on drugs there remains considerable flexibility in consumption patterns. Addicted users typically consume more than they need to avoid withdrawal symptoms (Moore, 1977; Roumasset and Hadreas, 1977). Even 'regular users' do not consume drugs every day of the year (Moore, 1977; Hartnoll and Lewis, 1984). Changes in dependent users' consumption levels could occur for a number of reasons, such as increased prices or increases in the other costs of obtaining drugs. White and Luksetich (1983) emphasized that there were many options available to dependent drug users faced with increased costs of use: decreased frequency of use; a change in the drug of choice; quit drug use altogether; continued use at a higher level of cost or entry into treatment. Thus, even the consumption patterns of dependent drug users will be affected by a wide range of influences.

There are many harms that are associated with dependent heroin use. Some of these problems are listed in Table 4.1 but, whilst many of these costs have been associated with drug use, not all of the harm can necessarily be attributed to that use. Dependent drug users will seek to avoid the 'costs' of drug withdrawal and may engage in crime to finance their habit. However, the association may not be a one-way relationship since Grapendaal (1992) discovered evidence that the level of drug use depends on available income, with many users celebrating receipt of money or successful crime with a purchase of drugs. Similarly, the findings of some fieldwork studies have suggested that criminal activity will continue even if drug use can be reduced or eliminated (Burr, 1987). There are analogous complications in the attribution of unemployment, mental health problems and social dysfunctioning to illicit heroin use. Nevertheless, drug use does cause considerable problems for some individuals, especially through overdoses. Determining the exact amount of individual harm for non-dependent users poses even greater problems, and even within dependent users there may be large variations in both the perceived and actual balance of costs and benefits from continued illicit drug use.

Economics rationalizes society's concerns about the use of illicit drugs in terms of the uncompensated costs (harms) imposed by drug use on third-parties (Culyer, 1973). Since illicit drug use may have effects on non-users, such as crime and HIV-transmission, society has a rationale for influencing the choices made by (potential) drug users. In addition, society may seek to change patterns of drug-use if addiction, peer-pressure, and the early age at which many drug-users begin using illicit drugs, are seen to be a departure from rational decision-making.

There are many harms associated with drug-use, which society may attempt to reduce. Crimes committed by drug users either to finance drug purchases as discussed above, as a result of intoxication, or in contractual disputes in the illicit market, produce obvious harms for victims, as well as an increased fear of crime for the rest of the community. Illicit drug markets themselves generate a range of harms, in the case of community concerns over visible drug dealing in certain areas (Gilman and Pearson, 1991), parental and familial concerns about others' drug use, and the fear of a 'contagion effect'. Premature death and increased

Table 4.1: Harms with which drug use is associated

Dimension	Type of harm
Crime	Committed under the influence
	Committed to buy drugs
	Disputes over drug market transactions
	Contacts made in criminal society
Health	Overdoses
	Accidents whilst under the influence
	HIV-risk
	Hepatitis B and C
	Poisoning through adulterants
	Abscesses, ulcers and sores
	Thrombosis
	Effects of drugs themselves
	Poor drug-using lifestyles
	Addiction
	Effects on babies' health
Employment/education	Qualifications obtained
	Jobs selection
	Chances of securing work
	Productivity and sickness absence
Social	Pain and suffering of friends/family
	Effect on local environment

Source: Chatterton *et al.* (1995).

morbidity will impose costs on society in terms of productivity losses and society's valuations of human life and poor health status. In addition, illicit drug use may cause educational under-achievement, truancy, and employment problems. Furthermore, substance misuse will have resource implications for other public policies, in the form of additional social security payments, police and other Criminal Justice System costs of crimes caused by drug use, as well as medical costs in Accident and Emergency Departments.

Costs and Benefits to Individuals of Methadone Maintenance Programmes

Different treatments will involve both the user and society in a different pattern of costs and benefits. For the user, different interventions may involve greater personal costs or changes in lifestyle, and these costs may affect their retention in the treatment system.

Methadone is prescribed to dependent heroin users to offer relief from the withdrawal consequences of abstaining from heroin. The drug is of relatively low potency compared to other opiates, is normally taken orally (as opposed to injected), and has a long half-life thereby delaying withdrawal symptoms (Raistrick *et al.*, 1995). Within the spectrum of illicit drug treatments, methadone was traditionally used to aid the user to attain a drug-free state. Doses of methadone were traditionally supplied on a reducing dose basis and for a relatively short time period (Franey *et al.*, 1993). Few services were prepared to consider maintenance therapy, i.e. the supply of methadone with no agreed timetable for reducing and eliminating doses, although clinical freedom has allowed a wide variety of prescribing practices to develop. However, the growth of heroin use, concern about drug-use and HIV, along with evidence on the effectiveness of methadone maintenance therapy has increased the number of treatment agencies and general practitioners who are prescribing methadone to drug users.

For the individual, methadone prescription may offer a range of costs and benefits. According to Senay (1985), methadone maintenance therapy offers benefits ranging from a suppression of opioid-abstinence symptoms and a resultant relief from the need to commit crime, to an opportunity to initiate a therapeutic relationship which facilitates delivery of other care services. A more recent issue that has affected the provision of drug services is HIV-transmission. This is mainly seen in the provision of needle exchange schemes, but methadone maintenance is seen as a way of maintaining contact with drug users, and hence influencing their behaviour.

A range of costs to the individual can also be considered. Tangible costs faced by treatment clients include the time and travel costs required for appointments and pick-up of prescriptions from the pharmacy – some methadone maintenance treatments involve a daily collection of scripts. Fears about addiction to another drug, and more severe and protracted withdrawal pains associated with methadone, have been reported (Watson, 1985; Burr, 1989; Grapendaal, 1992). Any reduced need to purchase heroin on the illicit market may reduce the need to commit crime for some users, but may increase the disposable income of others and may encourage the purchase of other illicit drugs or alcohol (Chatterton *et al.*, 1995).

Many programmes do not expect clients to reduce illicit drug use to zero, and low-threshold services (which offer low doses of methadone and little client–worker contact) have been suggested to be an important condition for the continuation of a drug-using lifestyle for some users (Grapendaal, 1992). A more confrontational approach to clients' drug use than is offered by maintenance prescriptions may be beneficial to some. There is some evidence on this possibility based on the only randomized controlled trial of heroin prescription conducted in the mid-1970s. In the more confrontational arm of the trial (in this case methadone maintenance), more subjects became abstinent and more continued to have severe problems, than in the heroin prescription arm (Hartnoll *et al.*, 1980). With the current provision of services, methadone maintenance may be a less confrontational option in comparison to rapid detoxification. Some heroin users who do not contact services or are forced to wait for treatment may be more likely to attempt and achieve non-medicated rapid detoxification. Methadone maintenance offers benefits relative to dependent illicit heroin use, but may be judged worse than complete abstinence. It is feasible that the provision of methadone maintenance therapy reduces the probability of abstinence in the short-term.

Detoxification following maintenance therapy is an important issue. Cushman's (1981) review of follow-up study results indicated very high rates of relapse to illicit opiate use in detoxed methadone maintenance patients – in a follow-up of 17000 individuals who had been prescribed methadone only 8 per cent were apparently well. The detoxification procedure is relatively straightforward, but many patients relapse because they are exposed to opiates again (Lowinson, 1981). In addition, methadone maintenance patients cannot expect to be opiate-free in the short-term – the journey from methadone to abstinence is described as 'an 18 to 24 month term treatment concept, heterogeneously applied' (Cushman, 1981, p. 391). Of course, the likelihood and continued success of detoxification depends on the individual, the individual's circumstances, and the reasons for seeking detoxification. Unsurprisingly, those patients who break the rules of the treatment regime are the least likely to discontinue opiate use, and independent predictors of detoxification success are steady employment, social life outside the circle of drug-using friends, and length of time in treatment (with chances of success increasing significantly after three years) (Cushman, 1981).

Costs and Benefits to Society of Methadone Maintenance Programmes

The societal consequences of methadone maintenance programmes may be the primary concern of policy-makers. In arguing for methadone maintenance therapy, the justification has frequently been in terms of addressing society rather than individual drug users' concerns (Lowinson, 1981). Individuals stabilized on methadone and in regular contact with treatment services have been found to have improved health, reduced criminal activity and reduced levels of illicit drug use (Senay, 1985; Ball and Ross, 1991; Farrell *et al.*, 1994). In the United States, a number of studies on the relative magnitudes of social cost savings (usually in terms of reduced crime and increased productivity of treated drug users) and the resource inputs required have found methadone programmes to be highly cost-beneficial (Des Jarlais *et al.*, 1981; Tabbush, 1986; Harwood *et al.*, 1988; Gerstein *et al.*, 1994; Rydell and Everingham, 1994).

The applicability of these findings to decisions about whether to expand services is not clear. In most cases the results refer to individuals who have voluntarily entered treatment. As individuals' perceptions change to negative testimonies about their drug use (Gilman and Pearson, 1991), it is feasible that a decision is also made to quit crime. For example, in Ball and Ross's (1991) analysis of reductions in criminality resulting from methadone maintenance programmes, the greatest proportion of crime reduction occurred in the short time-period before treatment entry. Randomized controlled trials of methadone maintenance therapy indicate that individual motivation is not an explanation for all of the benefits that accrue to treatment-attending clients (Farrell *et al.*, 1994). Nevertheless, there have been very few studies of individuals who have reached the same stage in their drug-using career and not been able to gain access to treatment (see Watson, 1985, for an exception).

Little attention seems to have been paid to evaluating possible costs that methadone maintenance may impose on society. For example, in the literature, authors rarely analyse the direct costs of providing services. A recent costing study estimated that, over the study period of a year, the average cost of care for an outpatient opiate client was £840 (Coyle *et al.*, 1994). The provision of methadone maintenance services has high opportunity costs in terms of alternative care which could be provided with these resources. For example, it is obvious that non-medicated detoxification is cheaper than methadone-based withdrawal (Caplehorn and Saunders, 1993).

An alternative source of cost that may be placed on society is through 'leakage'. Few services in Britain supervise the administration of oral methadone. As a result, prescribed methadone may be sold on the illicit market to users attempting to self-medicate. If self-medication of methadone offers some benefits to society or individuals in terms of a reduced need for illicit heroin, this may be seen as an extension of treatment services, and the optimal level of leakage may not be zero (Reuter, 1994). Alternatively, methadone may be taken inappropriately, in conjunction with alcohol or by non drug-using third parties, raising the risk of overdose.

Finally, methadone maintenance may increase the harm caused to society if there is a significant effect on the illicit market and/or the size of the drug-using population. It has been argued above that methadone prescription may reduce the probability, in some cases, of abstinence and increase the length of the drug-using career. It is possible, therefore, for methadone prescriptions to increase the size of the illicit heroin market. From society's perspective, reduction of the size of the drug-using population may be seen as the major aim of policy.

Unintended behaviour consequences have been considered in evaluations of needle exchange facilities. Guydish *et al.* (1993) considered whether the introduction of a needle exchange had increased injecting drug use, increased needle-sharing, or encouraged drug users to switch from non-injection to injection. However, measurement of the prevalence of illicit drug use and the monitoring of drug-use behaviour is notoriously difficult (Institute for the Study of Drug Dependence, 1992; Sutton and Maynard, 1992; Shapiro, 1993). Guydish *et al.* (1993) relied on data obtained from individuals attending the needle exchange, with obvious problems of selection bias. Nevertheless, the results indicate that some negative effects may occur (such as an increase in the frequency of injection with greater availability of needles), although these changes were judged to be insignificant in relation to trends in behaviour shortly before the study period.

Ethical Rules for Trading-off Societal and Individual Level Costs and Benefits

Given the likelihood that conflicts will exist between the effects of drug treatments on individuals and on society, at least in some circumstances, ethical judgements will be important in determining the treatment offered. Since methadone maintenance is provided by clinicians, it is likely that trade-offs between individual and societal levels are currently made according to medical ethics. As summarized by Mooney (1992), the British Medical Association's *Handbook of Medical Ethics* emphasizes that a doctor's role in considering the allocation of resources is subordinate to their duty to do the best they can for the person who has sought treatment. A decision rule based on these values would follow a course of action dictated by the clinician's prediction of the balance of costs and benefits to the individual. The resultant costs and benefits to society would be considered only if the proposed course of action does no harm and no good to the individual. Clinicians, therefore, would be little concerned about any negative effects of methadone prescription on society, if it offers the individual the possibility of stability. Conversely, societal justifications for methadone therapy in terms of reductions in crime would be judged irrelevant if any harm was possible to the individual, or even if the intervention was believed to offer few benefits.

One economic approach to the problem of these trade-offs is *cost-benefit analysis*. In an economic evaluation the total value of the costs of providing methadone maintenance would be compared to the sum of the values of the benefits of this service. A first approximation to the resolution of these trade-offs is provided by the Hicks-Kaldor criterion. Under this decision rule, a policy change is judged to increase efficiency if it is possible for those who gained to compensate those who have lost out, and still be better off than before. As Friedman (1985, p. 164) states, 'it is critically important that the compensations are not in fact made'. It can be shown that this decision rule is anti-egalitarian, since gains to a person who is less well-off are judged to be socially *less* worthwhile than gains to a person who is better off (ibid, p. 171–2).

As many economists have not been content with this implication of the Hicks-Kaldor criterion, a two-stage process has been proposed. The identification, measurement and valuation of costs and benefits, and their distribution across different groups, represents the first stage. In a second stage these figures are presented to policy-makers for them to make these equity trade-offs more explicit, or otherwise alternative equity decision rules are proposed. Two such decision rules, which are thought to represent the two extremes of the acceptable range (Friedman, 1985), are Benthamite and Rawlsian equity criterion. Under a Benthamite decision rule, gains or losses are proposed to be equally worthwhile to society regardless of the group(s) upon which they impact. Under a Rawlsian alternative, the objective of social policy is to improve the situation of the least well-off, possibly at the expense of other groups who could receive benefits of a far greater magnitude.

Concern over the equity aspects of valuing life has led some economists to adopt alternative 'cost-utility' methods for health care interventions (Williams, 1994). While other costs and benefits are measured in the same way as in cost-benefit analysis, any loss of life or ill-health is measured in other units, such as the Quality-Adjusted Life Year. These units are generally taken to be of equal value to all individuals, whatever their age or wealth. Generally, however, these methods have been used when the individual undergoing treatment bears the major effects of the intervention.

The implications of these ethical decision rules for the provision of treatment depend on whether (potential) clients for drug treatment services are seen as the worst-off in society. Medical ethics treats societal impacts as subordinate to those at individual level. A Rawlsian ethical rule adopts a similar approach if clients are judged to be the worst-off in society. In these cases, methadone maintenance, for example, would be widely adopted only if there were clear demonstrable benefits to the individual. Other decision rules trade-off societal and individual impacts, some paying no attention to the relative position of the groups affected. These decision rules could lead to adoption of the intervention even if individuals derived little benefit.

A further complication is that clinical decisions may be based on individuals' health or drug-using status. Recommended evaluation instruments indicate that benefits and costs accrue over many dimensions, and that health benefits represent only a subset of the criteria over which treatment decisions will impact (Darke *et al.*, 1992). Currently, treatment services are funded in the main by the health care sector, particularly in the prescription of substitute drugs. However, if methadone maintenance is a method of reducing crime it will be of interest to the criminal justice system both as a 'preventive' measure and to be used as an alternative to custodial sentences. Given the present structure of decision-making and funding, however, criminal justice agencies have little scope for altering the level of treatment facilities in order to achieve reductions in the social costs of crime.

Conclusions

Public provision of services to improve the well-being of certain individuals will always involve trade-offs with other possible uses of these resources. In the case of treatments for drug problems, there are also likely to be more complex trade-offs between individual and societal effects; impacts on the drug-using population and the rest of society; and even within the drug-using population. Some examples of possible conflicts between different groups have been indicated in this chapter for the case of methadone maintenance therapy, but other ethical problems will arise for other treatment options, and for the prevention or enforcement approaches.

Drug treatments, and methadone maintenance programmes in particular, will remain a controversial treatment until more data on the impact of treatment on the individual and society are available. These data may indicate that there are net gains for a group of current heroin users and society as a whole. Future programmes that aim to match variations in methadone therapies to patient groups may help minimize the costs to individuals and maximize benefits to society, but have not as yet been fully evaluated (Raistrick *et al.*, 1995). Such findings may avoid the potential ethical conflicts outlined in this paper, but would not necessarily result in an efficient level of funding given the non-health benefits that may accrue. Evaluations that suggest substantial gains for society but more equivocal results on the value of this intervention for individuals could raise considerable conflicts across different professional groups. Economic analysis is one means of making trade-offs between groups explicit, but cannot 'solve' these ethical issues.

References

BALL, J.C. and ROSS, A. (1991) *The Effectiveness of Methadone Maintenance Treatment*, New York: Springer-Verlag.

BURR, A. (1987) 'Chasing the dragon', *British Journal of Criminology*, **27**, 4, pp. 333–57.

BURR, A. (1989) 'An inner-city community response to heroin-use', in McGREGOR, S. (Ed.) *Drugs and British Society*, Routledge: London.

CAPLEHORN, J.R.M. and SAUNDERS, J.B. (1993) 'A comparison of residential heroin detoxification patients and methadone maintenance patients', *Drug and Alcohol Review*, **12**, pp. 259–63.

CHATTERTON, M., GIBSON, G., GILMAN, M., GODFREY, C., SUTTON, M. and WRIGHT, A. (1995) *Performance Indicators for Local Anti-Drugs Strategies – A Preliminary Analysis*, Police Paper 62, Police Research Group. London: Home Office Police Department.

COYLE, D., GODFREY, C., HARDMAN, G. and RAISTRICK, D. (1994) *Costing Substance Misuse Services*, Yorkshire Addictions Research, Training and Information

Consortium (YARTIC) Occasional Paper 5, York: Centre for Health Economics, University of York.

CULYER, A. (1973) 'Should social policy concern itself with drug abuse?', *Public Finance Quarterly*, **1**, 4, pp. 449–56.

CUSHMAN, P. (1981) 'Detoxification after methadone treatment', in LOWINSON, J.H. and RUIZ, P. (Eds) *Substance Abuse: Clinical Problems and Perspectives*, Baltimore: Williams and Wilkins.

DARKE, S., HALL, W., WODAK, A., HEATHER, N. and WARD, J. (1992) 'Development and validation of a multi-dimensional instrument for assessing outcome of treatment among opiate users: the Opiate Treatment Index', *British Journal of Addiction*, **87**, pp. 733–42.

DES JARLAIS, D., DEREN, S. and LIPTON, D.S. (1981) 'Cost effectiveness studies in the evaluation of substance abuse treatment', in LOWINSON, J.H. and RUIZ, P. (Eds) *Substance Abuse: Clinical Problems and Perspectives*, Baltimore: William and Wilkins.

FARRELL, M., WARD, J., MATTICK, R., HALL, W., STIMSON, G.V. DES JARLAIS, D., GOSSOP, M. and STRANG, J. (1994) 'Methadone maintenance treatment in opiate dependence: a review', *British Medical Journal*, **309**, pp. 997–1001.

FRANEY, C., POWER, R. and WELLS, B. (1993) 'Treatment and services for drug users in Britain', *Journal of Substance Abuse Treatment*, **10**, pp. 561–7.

FRIEDMAN, L.S. (1985) *Microeconomic Policy Analysis*, New York: McGraw-Hill.

GERSTEIN, D.R., JOHNSON, R.A., HARWOOD, H., FOUNTAIN, D., SUTER, N. and MALLOY, K. (1994) *Evaluating recovery services: the California Drug and Alcohol Treatment Assessment (CALDATA)*, State of California: Community WORKS – Treatment, Department of Alcohol and Drug Programs.

GILMAN, M. and PEARSON, G. (1991) 'Lifestyles and law enforcement', in WHYNES, D.K. and BEAN, P.T. (Eds) *Policing and Prescribing*, London: MacMillan, pp. 95–124.

GRAPENDAAL, M. (1992) 'Cutting their coat according to their cloth: economic behaviour of Amsterdam opiate users', *The International Journal of the Addictions*, **27**, 4, pp. 487–501.

GUYDISH, J., BUCARDO, J., YOUNG, M., WOODS, W., GRINSTEAD, O. and CLARK, W. (1993) 'Evaluating needle exchange: are there negative effects?', *AIDS*, **7**, pp. 871–6.

HARTNOLL, R.L., MITCHESON, M.C., BATTERSBY, A., BROWN, G., ELLIS, M., FLEMING, P. and HEDLEY, N. (1980) 'Evaluation of heroin maintenance in controlled trial', *Archives of General Psychiatry*, **37**, pp. 877–84.

HARTNOLL, R. and LEWIS, R. (1984) *The illicit heroin market in Britain: towards a preliminary estimate of national demand*, Mimeo: Drugs Indicator Project, London: University College of London.

HARWOOD, H.J., HUBBARD, R.L., COLLINS, J.J. and RACHAL, J.V. (1988) *The costs of crime and the benefits of drug abuse treatment: a cost-benefit analysis using TOPS data*, NIDA Research Monograph; 86, pp. 209–35.

HOME OFFICE (1990) *UK Action on Drug Misuse: The Government's Strategy*, London: Home Office.

INSTITUTE FOR THE STUDY OF DRUG DEPENDENCE (1992) *Drug Misuse in Britain: national audit of drug misuse statistics*, London: ISDD.

LOWINSON, J.H. (1981) 'Methadone maintenance in perspective', in LOWINSON, J.H. and RUIZ, P. (Eds) *Substance Abuse: Clinical Problems and Perspectives*, Baltimore: Williams and Wilkins.

MOONEY, G. (1992) *Economics, Medicine and Health Care*, 2nd Edn., London: Harvester-Wheatsheaf.

MOORE, M.H. (1977) *Buy and Bust*, Lexington, USA: D.C. Heath and Company.

RAISTRICK, D., GODFREY, C., HAY, A., SUTTON, M., TOBER, G. and WOOLF, K. (1995) *Prescribing methadone*, Yorkshire Addictions Research, Training and Information Consortium (YARTIC) Occasional Paper 7, York: Centre for Health Economics, University of York.

REUTER, P. (1994) 'Identifying new policy trade-offs', *Addiction*, **89**, 7, pp. 806.

ROUMASSET, J. and HADREAS, J. (1977) 'Addicts, fences, and the market for stolen goods', *Public Finance Quarterly*, **5**, 2, pp. 247–72.

RYDELL, C.P. and EVERINGHAM, S.S. (1994) *Controlling Cocaine: supply versus demand programs*, California: Drug Policy Research Center, RAND.

SENAY, E.C. (1985) 'Methadone maintenance treatment', *International Journal of the Addictions*, **20**, 6 and 7, pp. 803–821.

SHAPIRO, H. (1993) 'Where does all the snow go? The prevalence and pattern of cocaine and crack use in Britain', in BEAN, P. (Ed.) *Cocaine and Crack: Supply and Use*, Basingstoke: MacMillan.

SUTTON, M. and MAYNARD, A. (1992) *What is the size and nature of the 'drug problem' in the UK?*, Yorkshire Addictions Research, Training and Information Consortium (YARTIC) Occasional Paper 3, York: Centre for Health Economics, University of York.

SUTTON, M. and MAYNARD, A. (1994) *Trends in the cost-effectiveness of drug enforcement activity in the illicit heroin market 1979–1990*. Yorkshire Addictions Research, Training and Information Consortium (YARTIC) Occasional Paper 4, York: Centre for Health Economics and Leeds Addiction Unit.

TABBUSH, V. (1986) *The effectiveness and efficiency of publicly funded drug abuse treatment and prevention programs in California: a benefit-cost analysis*, California: University of California Press.

WATSON, P. (1985) *The Fate of Drug Addicts on a Waiting List*, England: Report to the North Western Regional Health Authority.

WILLIAMS, A. (1994) *Economics, QALYS and Medical Ethics: A Health Economist's Perspective*, Discussion Paper 121. York: Centre for Health Economics, University of York.

WHITE, M.D. and LUKSETICH, W.A. (1983) Heroin: price elasticity and enforcement strategies, *Economic Inquiry*, **21**, pp. 557–564.

Chapter 5

Means-Testing for Social Assistance: UK Policy in an International Perspective[1]

Tony Eardley

Introduction

Welfare benefits allocated on the basis of a test of resources are attracting increasing international interest. The number of people claiming resource-tested 'safety net' benefits has been increasing in many developed countries in Europe and beyond, as a consequence of growing long-term unemployment (especially amongst young people), rises in lone parenthood and other social changes. Population ageing and global economic competitiveness are also putting pressure on the financing of insurance based social security schemes and non-contributory categorical benefits – fuelling calls for some benefits to be subjected to income- or means-testing.

The principle of determining support for people in need according to the resources already available to them has a long history – indeed it can be seen as the fundamental corner stone of the Poor Laws, which pre-dated current social security systems across Europe. The application of means tests has changed considerably since the abandonment of the harsh and deterrent regimes of the workhouse and the later but no less unpopular 'household means test' of 1930s Britain. Nevertheless, resource-testing continues to involve a series of administrative decisions about what constitutes the private resources of a benefit applicant; with whom these resources are assumed to be shared; who in a family or household should be expected to contribute personal resources to the upkeep of other individuals; and how much of the available private resources should be consumed before there is a call on public assistance. What can often be seen as technical decisions are in fact questions of policy, even of morality and ideology, reflecting wider attitudes towards the balance of responsibilities between the state and the individual or family. For example, if older retired people apply for benefit, should their adult children be asked to contribute to their upkeep? If they own a house that is larger than their current needs, should they be expected to sell it before being able to claim assistance? How far should claimants have to consume their savings before benefit is available and what message does this convey about thrift? At what point and under what circumstances should a man involved in a relationship with a lone mother be assumed to be responsible for her financial upkeep? All of these are important and difficult questions which an assistance scheme has to address. The structure of any resource-tested benefit is also inevitably linked with questions of work incentives or other possible behavioural effects, either implicitly or, as is increasingly the case, quite explicitly. Thus, taking into account all part-time earnings of unemployed claimants may be counter-productive (especially for couples) if it provides no incentive for them to increase their earnings through extra work, but taken too far, a policy of disregarding earnings can create disincentive effects of its own.

The potential for variation in these different dimensions of the resource-testing process is therefore considerable. Many different structures could be envisaged, which would still fall within the general description of a 'means test'. Indeed, even within the UK, where a common structure for the main means-tested benefits has existed since 1988, there are still significant differences between the rules applying to the basic benefit for the unemployed (Income Support) and those for Family Credit, which is designed for families in low-paid work. Also, under new arrangements for the financing of community care local authorities are assessing resources in a variety of ways to determine access to and charges for local services (Lunt and Corden, 1996 forthcoming).

The United Kingdom has one of the most extensive national systems of means-tested benefits in the world. Nearly 16 per cent of the total population, including about a quarter of all children aged under 16 were supported through Income Support alone in 1992/3. Around half a million families currently receive Family Credit, while millions of other individuals and families get means-tested help with housing and council tax payments. The most recent addition to the armoury of resource-tested benefits is Disability Working Allowance, for disabled people in low-paid part-time work. The UK, however, is not alone in operating resource-tested systems for securing a minimum level of cash income for people without sufficient other means. Most developed countries have some form of social 'safety net' available to part, if not all, of their populations. How far are their policies on means-testing similar or different to those of the UK and what are the sources and implications of different policy approaches? The answer to this question is important, particularly if the use of means-testing is expanding, because it helps us to distinguish between approaches that appear to be inevitable and intrinsic to the nature of means-testing and those which may be culturally or politically driven.

This chapter outlines and discusses different approaches to resource testing for social assistance in the countries that are members of the Organization for

Tony Eardley

Economic Co-operation and Development (OECD), drawing on a study of assistance schemes in 24 countries. The chapter begins by briefly reviewing the reasons for the increase of interest in selectivity through resource testing, and then attempts to clarify some of the terminology involved. The next section describes the key features of means-testing for benefits in the UK. This is then put in an international context by comparing the UK with other OECD countries. A concluding section discusses the implications of the different approaches.

The Growth of Interest in Means-Testing

Arguments in favour of selectivity in benefit delivery on the basis of claimants' resources appear to have been gaining ground internationally in recent years. The perception that a level of social security expenditure which requires relatively high taxation and employer costs may damage economic effort, particularly in the context of global competition, has become increasingly dominant in international political and economic discourse. This perception has been forcefully expressed by the UK Government in negotiations with its EU partners on the social dimension of the Union. It is also a common thread that runs through the OECD's analyses of member countries' recent economic performance, as well through the Jobs Study, which examined unemployment and proposed strategies for coping with labour market change (Organization for Economic Co-operation and Development, 1994). Whilst the European Commission and many of the EU governments have resisted any wholesale reduction of insurance based social protection, the White Paper on Growth, Competitiveness and Employment (Commission of the European Communities, 1994) recommends a range of measures aimed at increasing employment, which include reductions in employers' non-wage costs and boosting of work incentives through income related supplements to earnings.

The general economic arguments for greater 'targeting' are well known. In particular, benefits targeted on those most in need may be more effective and efficient at closing poverty gaps than universal payments, which may go in part to people who do not need them (Beckerman, 1979). In times of economic stringency, the idea that poverty can be more effectively alleviated by reallocating existing transfers is attractive. On an international level, targeting is seen as the most effective tool, as suggested by the World Bank's 1990 World Development Report, which stated that:

> ... a comprehensive approach to poverty reduction calls for a program
> of well-targeted transfers and safety nets as an essential complement to
> the basic strategy. (World Bank, 1990, p. 3; quoted in Atkinson, 1993)

In line with this strategy, economic aid from the international financial institutions (including the World Bank and the International Monetary Fund) to the transitional economies of Eastern Europe has also increasingly been weighted towards the establishment of means-tested 'safety nets' to back-up limited insurance based systems. Within the European Union, one response to research suggesting high levels of poverty amongst its citizens (for a discussion of which see Room, 1990) has been to adopt a Draft Recommendation (Commission of the European Communities, 1991), urging member countries to institute guarantees of minimum resources based primarily on the assistance model.

The drawbacks of the targeted approach are also well known (see for example, Deacon and Bradshaw, 1983; Saunders, 1991; Atkinson, 1992; Gough, 1994): they include potential problems of poverty traps, intrusive enquiry and stigma; low take-up; social divisiveness; and high administrative costs. There is also a danger in concentrating on poverty relief to the exclusion of other possible legitimate objectives for social security. A further argument is that focusing benefits on the poor may undermine the wider support for social security which is needed to finance effective targeted schemes (Saunders, 1991). Overall, there is a general problem of whether targets themselves are adequately defined, and whether policy instruments can be designed accurately enough to hit them (Whiteford, 1994).

The arguments for and against targeting are often presented at a level of principle which assumes that all forms of means-testing are alike. In fact, there are important distinctions. Some Australian social policy analysts, for example, have questioned the generalized critiques of targeting which stem particularly from a 'Nordo-centric' emphasis on equality through universal benefits (Mitchell, 1991; Mitchell *et al.*, 1994). They have argued, from the perspective of the almost entirely resource-tested Australian social security system, that it is the outcomes of different policy arrangements that are important rather than the instruments, and that targeting is not a policy which intrinsically leads to greater inequality.

Conceptual issues in means-testing for social assistance

The first problem in discussing means-testing in this context arises from the definition of the term 'social assistance'. It is not a term with a precise definition internationally, especially in translation. In some countries, particularly those of the Nordic group, social assistance is a concept associated not only with income maintenance but also with social work service, and individual treatment or rehabilitation. In some other countries, it is understood as referring mainly to discretionary supplementary schemes that are subsidiary to the main means-tested minimum income benefit. Taking branches of social security or benefits simply by their names may be misleading – one reason why Brown *et al.* (1991) have suggested abandoning the term social assistance altogether in comparative studies. What is being referred to here is the range of benefits available to guarantee a minimum (however defined) level of subsistence to people in need, based on a test of resources. However, even this definition is not without problems, as there are countries where minimum income protection for some groups of people, particularly those over retirement age or disabled, comes through non-contributory 'citizens' benefits or pensions awarded without a test of other resources.

A further difficulty arises in respect of benefits that *are* tested against applicants' resources, but are designed to exclude higher earners rather than to offer a guaranteed minimum to the lowest income groups. There are examples of these in several countries, and they often derive from the selective refocussing of benefits, such as family allowances that were previously universal. There are several other distinctions, and it helps at this point to introduce a taxonomy of means-tested benefits developed for the purposes of the social assistance study.

The first distinction is between those benefits aimed at providing a minimum 'safety net', below which people's current income should not fall (we call this 'poverty-tested'), and others which relate benefits to resources across a wider range of income. The first benefits are what we normally think of as 'social assistance' and the second might be described as 'selective' benefits. The second division is between cash benefits for general use and 'tied' benefits, which could be in kind or in the form of services, or alternatively may be linked to reductions in the cost of specified goods or services. (This would include housing benefits.) The third partition is between those benefits available to all people within a particular income or resources group and those only for specified categories of people within this group. These categorizations generate the model in Table 5.1.

Even within this approach, absolute consistency cannot be achieved, because in some countries there are important benefits that are resource-tested and available in full when other income is very low, but which are withdrawn at a rate of less than 100 per cent as other income increases – often tapering out

Table 5.1: A taxonomy of means testing

		All Groups	Specific Groups
Social assistance	Cash	1	2
	Tied	3	4
Selective	Cash	5	6
	Tied	7	8

Source: Gough (1994), modified

at a considerably higher level of income than would allow entitlement to the main social assistance benefit. The UK's Family Credit is a prime example. Such benefits are important because, to extend the circus analogy, they are intended to act less as 'safety nets' and more as trampolines or springboards to help lift beneficiaries back into independence through labour market participation.

In practice, categorizing all the assorted means-tested schemes in operation in the 24 countries of the study is not at all easy. The distinction between 'poverty-tested' social assistance and some other selective schemes that go a little further up the income scale is not always clear cut. Nor is the distinction between cash and 'tied' benefits always apparent; especially in schemes such as Canada's where housing allowances are paid as part of the assistance calculation and are not necessarily related to actual rent paid. For the purposes of this chapter, and in order to help illustrate some of the differences in approach, even within benefit systems that have the most in common, the analysis is restricted mainly to schemes which provide cash assistance at the minimum level; either to all groups or at least to a substantial number of categories of people in a broadly similar way (cells 1 and 2 in the model, Table 5.1). The main benchmark for comparison is the UK's Income Support scheme.

A final problem of terminology concerns the use of 'means-tested', 'income-tested' or 'income-related', and 'asset-tested' to refer to different forms of resource-testing. The terms are sometimes used in the literature loosely or interchangeably, but they do have different meanings, even if the processes which they are describing are not always clear cut. Here, income-tested or income-related benefits are taken to be those where the level of benefit to which a claimant is entitled is based only on an assessment of his or her earnings or other income (however defined) and where capital or other property and assets are not taken into account. Some benefits have specific rules relating to the value of property or other assets that applicants may have, and still be entitled to benefit, and these are described as assets tests. Where both income and assets are taken into account benefits are described as means-tested. This definition of means-testing encompasses those benefits where there are no specific limits to the amount of capital or savings an applicant can have, but where savings are deemed to produce a notional amount of weekly or monthly income, which is then counted in the income test.

Means-Testing for Social Assistance in the UK

It was stated earlier that resource-testing is based on a series of decisions about the resource unit, the members of the family or household who might be expected to contribute to a claimant's maintenance, and the sources and amounts of income or assets taken into account. Income Support is means-tested according to our definition, since it is subject to both income and capital limits and savings are deemed to generate a specified amount of income.[2] The 'benefit unit' (those people covered by an individual claim) consists of the claimant, a spouse if there is one and any dependent children (subject to a set of regulations defining dependency). Thus, it basically coincides with the nuclear family. Other non-dependent adults living in the household, such as the claimant's grown-up children, siblings or parents, are treated as separate benefit units if they have the need to claim Income Support. In the case of a couple, either partner may claim for the whole benefit unit. Payment is then made to the person who has made the claim. There are no general administrative facilities for splitting payments, although this can happen in exceptional circumstances, such as where a claimant has an alcohol problem and may spend his or her benefit on drink.

The 'resource unit' – those members of the family or household whose resources may be assessed in the means-test, and who thus may be expected to contribute to the maintenance of the benefit unit – is also the nuclear family. Where two people (of the opposite sex) live together they are treated as cohabiting, and thus part of the same benefit and resource unit, if the evidence shows that they live together 'as man and wife'. The key difference between the benefit and resource unit, however, is that the assumption of a degree of resource sharing applies to some non-dependent adults in a claimant's household, and a set of standard deductions are made from the housing cost element of a claimant's benefit entitlement according to the circumstances of the non-dependant. Thus, for example, a young person above the age of 'dependency' but still living with her or his parents is assumed to be making a contribution towards the housekeeping. These deductions have been increased over the years and are not insubstantial. In 1995/6, the deduction for an adult aged 18 or more in full-time work, for example, is between £5 and £30 per week, depending on the level of their gross income. This means that the presence of a non-dependant earning £145 per week or more in the household of a couple with one child aged 10 would result in a reduction of housing support (either through Income Support mortgage interest payments or Housing Benefit) equivalent to 30 per cent of their basic benefit entitlement.

Most income of the benefit unit is taken into account in full in the means test, including other social security benefits, with the exception of certain benefits that compensate for additional costs for disabled people, certain war pensions and some earnings. Spouse and child maintenance payments are counted in full for Income Support (though partial disregards now exist for some other means-tested benefits). Child benefit and one parent benefit are also counted in full.

Earnings are taken into account after the deduction of any income tax and national insurance contributions, and half of any contributions towards a pension. Since April 1988 it has not been possible to offset work expenses (travel-to-work, child care) before earnings are taken into account. A small amount of earnings are disregarded. For Income Support this is £5 per week per individual or per member of a couple, but a higher disregard of £15 applies to lone parents; couples under 60 who have been receiving income support for two years or more; carers receiving the carers' premium; single people or couples entitled to the disability premium or higher pensioner premium; and a few categories of reserve/emergency workers. Children's earnings and other income are usually wholly disregarded, and even when included only count against the benefit payable for that child. Special rules apply to childminders' earnings, and to income from subtenants and lodgers. For childminders, only one third of earnings is counted as income after deducting any tax and national insurance.

Assets are usually taken to include cash, money held in accounts, and the net market value of land or property (except a dwelling owned and occupied by the claimant as his/her home). Capital held by couples is added together. The first £3000 of capital is ignored. Capital between £3000 and £8000 is taken into account by making a deduction from benefit of £1 for every £250 over £3000 (called a 'tariff income'). Capital of more than £8000 excludes the owner from Income Support entitlement altogether. The value of personal possessions is usually ignored, as are certain forms of capital such as the surrender value of life insurance policies. Property that is not occupied is usually counted as capital, with some exceptions (including a six-month period when someone is trying to sell it). If dependent children have more than £3000 of capital their parents do not receive any benefit for them.

If someone is judged to have disposed of property or assets in order to be able to claim benefit, they are treated as still being in possession of that capital. This may result in exclusion from benefit, though a 'diminishing capital rule' should be applied, so that the exclusion is not indefinite. For Income Support, any income or increases in income over the prescribed level (after appropriate disregards) are taken into account pound for pound, that is at a withdrawal rate of 100 per cent.

Clearly, resource testing for the basic subsistence benefit in the UK has moved some way from the household means test of the 1930s and is now more in tune with the contemporary realities of family life and expectations. Nevertheless, substantial areas of controversy remain. The cohabitation rule, for example, which states that people of the opposite sex living together 'as man and wife' must be counted as part of the same benefit unit, is often seen as problematic in the context of contemporary lifestyles and ideas of the independence of women within relationships. It has led to intrusive surveillance and investigation of the lives of lone mothers, to see, for example, how many nights in a week a man friend stays over in the woman's dwelling. It has also been pointed out that the treatment of cohabitants within social security is inconsistent – recognising cohabitation only where it would restrict entitlement, as in Income Support, but not, as in contributory benefits, where it would grant the unmarried partner rights (Kiernan and Estaugh, 1993). The problems of abolishing the cohabitation rule and moving to a system of full independent rights to means-tested benefits, however, are also substantial, and this has been recognised by feminist critics of the current system as well (Lister, 1992). Abolishing the cohabitation rule could be very costly, since it might be difficult to justify not extending the same rights to married partners; it would involve a massive extension of means-testing; and it would tend to ignore the fact that resource sharing within couples does take place – even if not always on an equitable basis (Esam and Berthoud, 1991). These and other problems have led Lister (1992) among others to conclude that a strategy for women's access to independent income is not best pursued through means-tested benefits.

Another controversial issue, for lone parents in particular, is the counting in full of child maintenance in the means test; which one parent family organizations and other critics of the Child Support Agency have argued provides little incentive for women to claim maintenance or for men to pay it (Millar, 1994). Comparing the UK and Australian systems of child support, Millar and Whiteford (1993) calculated that in Australia in 1992 a lone parent on benefit (assessed as entitled to support from a former partner on average male earnings) would gain the equivalent of around £34 per week or almost 60 per cent of the child support, whereas in the UK she would gain nothing. The Government argument has been that the incentive structure is provided through Family Credit, within which there is now a partial maintenance disregard, and that a similar disregard in Income Support could simply trap lone parents on benefit.

One further longstanding argument has been about the low level of earnings disregards in Income Support, which tend to create disincentives for part-time work, particularly for the spouses of unemployed claimants. For people with children, however, Family Credit is designed to provide an incentive structure by offering those able to work at least 16 hours per week a withdrawal rate of earnings above Income Support level of 70 per cent rather than 100 per cent, together with the maintenance disregard and (since October 1994) a child care disregard with a maximum net value of £28 per week. Otherwise the means test for the two benefits is similar, though, unlike for Income Support, payments of Family Credit are fixed for six months at a time, with no requirement for claimants to report changes in income between claims.

Means-testing in a Comparative Context

Having outlined the basic structure of means testing for social assistance in the UK and having briefly touched on some key outstanding issues, we can now begin to see how these compare with those of other countries. Table 5.2 lays out in a schematic and abbreviated way some of the main elements of the assessment process for entitlement to the main assistance benefits in the countries in our study. The table indicates the administrative framework for the various benefits, since the operation of different types of means-testing may be linked to whether benefits have a national, or regulated structure, or are assessed at the discretion of local authorities. Benefit and resource units are also shown.

One problem with comparing the operation of means tests involves making sense of the many and varying ways in which assets are treated and the forms and levels of income which are disregarded in the test of resources. As a simplified way of classifying the treatment of earned income, countries are divided into four categories:

1 those applying no disregard;
2 those applying a minimal earnings disregard (up to 15 per cent of the standard single person rate);
3 those applying a medium disregard (between 16 and 40 per cent);
4 and those applying a higher disregard (over 40 per cent).

It should be noted that these are approximate calculations, since disregards are often made up in different ways; apply only to earned or unearned income; or vary for different family types. Sometimes they are only available for limited periods or are reduced over time, and this is indicated in the table.

The treatment of assets is also complex. In order to provide a comparison it is presented in two parts. First countries are divided into two groups:

1 those which take all liquid assets into account, applying only a small disregard or none at all;
2 and those applying a higher disregard to capital.

Secondly they are partitioned according to whether they tend to disregard the value of a private dwelling, or might expect claimants to sell their homes before drawing on assistance. There is also variety in the range of other income, including social security benefits, which is counted or disregarded as income in different countries. As an indicator of approaches to one key area of policy of contemporary relevance in a number of countries, the table shows whether child maintenance is counted as income.

The sources of information provided in the table are mainly the replies to a pro forma questionnaire completed by senior officials in the relevant ministry or department in each of the countries, together with other details and commentary supplied by a network of academic informants. Details of the methodology of the study can be found in Eardley *et al.* (1995). Unless otherwise stated the information applies to the year 1994/5.

Benefit and resource units

The first point to note from Table 5.2 is that although many countries describe entitlement to benefit as 'individual' – that is, anyone can be assessed for benefit on the basis of their individual entitlement – the actual unit for whom benefit is

Table 5.2: Conditions of entitlement to the main assistance benefits in 23 OECD countries

Country	Benefits	Legal and administrative framework	Benefit Unit	Resource Unit	Treatment of Income*	Treatment of Assets* Capital	Treatment of Assets* Disregard home?	Child Maintenance counted?
Australia	All	National regulations and administration	Family	Family	4 (with taper) more for the unemployed and partly individualized (from 1995/6)	2	Yes	Yes but with disregard
Austria	Sozialhilfe	Provincial mainly Discretionary	Household (incl. grandparents)	Household	1	1	Yes, if not too large, but LAs can take a charge on the equity	Yes, but only towards a child's needs
Belgium	Revenu Minimum d'Existence	National regulations Local administration	Family	Family (but recoverable from others)	4 (but reduced after 1st year)	1	Yes	Yes in full
Canada	Canada Assistance Plan	National framework. Provincial regulations and administration	Family	Family	3 (but varies between provinces)	2	Yes	Yes in full
Denmark	Social Bistand	National regulations Local administration	Family (cohabitants separate)	Family (but not cohabitants)	4 (but discretionary)	2	Yes	Yes in full
Finland	Social assistance allowance	National regulations Local administration	Family	Family	3 (but discretionary)	1	Yes	Yes in full
France	Revenu Minimum d'Insertion	Complex national and local framework	Family	Family	3	2	Yes	Yes in full

Table 5.2: Continued

Germany	*Sozialhilfe*	National regulations Regional rates and administration	Family	Household (and recoverable outside)	3–4 depending on Länd	1	Yes	Yes in full
Iceland	*Financial Assistance*	Local administration and regulations, but much discretion	Family (cohabitants separate)	Family (but not cohabitants)	1	1	Yes	Yes in full
Ireland	12 schemes including *Supplementary Welfare Allowance/Unemployment assistance*	National regulations and administration	Family	Family	U–4 SWA–1	2	Yes	Yes in full
Italy	*Minimo vitale*	Local and discretionary	Varies, but normally family	Varies, but normally household	Discretionary but likely to be 1	1	Yes	Discretionary
Japan	*Livelihood Aid*	National regulations Local administration	Household	Household	Not known	1 (discretionary)	Yes, if not luxurious	Yes in full
Luxembourg	*Revenu Minimum Garanti*	National regulations Local administration	Household (with exceptions)	Household	3	2	Yes	No
Netherlands	*Algemene Bistand* and Unemployment assistance (**RW**)	National regulations Local administration	Family	Family	2	2	Only if below specified levels	No
New Zealand	All	National regulations and administration	Family	Family	4 (with taper)	2	Yes	Yes in full
Norway	*Social and Economic Assistance*	National framework Local discretion	Family (cohabitants separate)	Family (not cohabitants)	2 (mainly lone parents)	1	Yes, if reasonable	Yes in full (but partial disregard for Transitional Allowance)
Portugal	No general assistance Ten social minimum schemes	National regulations	Family	Family	1	1	Yes	Yes in full

Table 5.2: Continued

Country	Benefits	Legal and administrative framework	Benefit Unit*	Resource Unit	Treatment of Income*	Treatment of Assets*		Child Maintenance counted?
						Capital	Disregard home?	
Spain	Ingreso Mínimo de Inserción	National framework Regional and local regulations and discretion	Family (cohabitants separate)	Family	1	1	Yes	Yes in full
Sweden	Social Welfare Allowance	National framework Local discretion	Family	Family	1	1	No, if alternative housing can be found	Yes in full
Switzerland	Soziale Fürsorge	Cantonal and municipal discretion	Household	Household	1 (discretionary)	1 (discretionary)	Yes if disabled	Yes but discretionary
Turkey	Social assistance and solidarity	National regulations Local administration	Household	Household	1	1	Not known	Yes in full
UK	Income support	National regulations	Family	Family, but deductions for non-dependants	2 (but family credit adds taper effect)	2	Yes	Yes in full (but partial disregard for family credit)
USA	1. Aid to Families with Dependent Children	State	Family	Family	3	2	Yes	1. Yes, but with disregard. varies
	2. Foodstamps	Federal/State	Household	Household	4	2	Yes	
	3. General Assistance	State/County	Family	Family	varies by State	1–2 depending on State	Some can take a charge on the equity	
	4. Supplemental Security Income	Federal/State	Individual	Individual/family	4	2	Yes	

Note: Greece is not included here as there is neither a generalized social assistance scheme, nor substantial cover through categorical schemes

*Income
1 those applying no disregard
2 those applying a minimal earnings disregard (up to 15 per cent of the standard single person rate)
3 those applying a medium disregard (between 16 and 40 per cent)
4 those applying a higher disregard (over 40 per cent)

Assets
1 those which take all liquid assets into account, applying only a small disregard or none at all
2 those applying a higher disregard to capital

payable is still normally the claimant plus the spouse and the dependent children in the case of non-single households, ie. the nuclear family. Only Austria, Luxembourg, and Japan count other non-dependent adults in the household as part of the benefit unit (and thus include their needs in the calculation of benefit due), and in Luxembourg there are many exceptions to this rule.

The differences become more marked, however, when we look at the resource unit – that is, the range of people whose resources must be taken into account when applying the test of a claimant's means. Again, the majority of countries take into account only the resources of the claimant and their spouse if they have one. Generally the resources of dependent children are fully, or partly, exempted and if they are counted it is normally only against the amounts of benefit specifically payable in respect of the children. In the UK, as we have seen, non-dependant deductions from housing costs imply an assumption of resource sharing within the wider household, but the expectation of intra-family support does not extend beyond this point (except for child maintenance). However, there are a number of countries where expectations of family support extend further.

In Austria, Germany, Japan and Switzerland, social assistance claimants may be expected to seek support from parents or grandparents, or in the case of older claimants from children and grandchildren – and in Switzerland, potentially from other siblings even – before having recourse to public assistance. It is also of interest in this respect to note that in Switzerland there are no standardized means tests: benefits are assessed according to a detailed and individual investigation of both resources and needs, using standard household budgets as a template. In France, *aide sociale* for older people (though not the *Revenu Minimum d'Insertion*) is subject to a prior test of their (future) inheritors' means: monies paid can be reclaimed from these family members, or by first claim on any assets left on death. In Belgium too, regulations were recently introduced that oblige local authorities to seek to recover assistance payments from parents or adult children of claimants. How these rules work in practice varies considerably and social welfare workers often have the discretion not to apply them, but what these countries share in common is a strong tradition of family responsibility and obligation, backed up in several countries by a structure of civil law, which specify duties of intra-family maintenance that go beyond that of spouses or of parent and child.

At the other end of the spectrum are a small group of countries which do not place a maintenance or resource-sharing obligation even on cohabiting couples unless they are legally married. In Denmark and Norway, the resources of a man cohabiting with a lone parent are not taken into account as part of her resources for an assistance claim, although some expenses may be taken as shared, particularly housing costs. In Iceland and Spain too, cohabitants have to register as living together and sharing resources – a reversal of the more common situation – and in Iceland there is no duty of maintenance within cohabiting couples unless a child of the relationship is involved. Although in a few countries, including the Netherlands, there has been some debate about cohabitation in terms of the equivalence structure of payments, the subject seems to excite little of the kind of controversy that has periodically been a feature of the UK system, particularly in the case of lone parents. It should be acknowledged, however, that the local and discretionary nature of many schemes potentially allows greater scrutiny of individuals' circumstances than may be apparent from formal description of the systems, particularly in those countries where people have to register their place of residence. Policy concerns about lone parenthood and cohabitation are also likely to be influenced by the number and percentage of lone parents claiming assistance, which vary considerable between countries. Around 70 per cent of all lone parents in the UK receive Income Support – one of the highest proportions among the countries of the Organization for Economic Co-operation and Development.

Although no countries have gone as far as general individualization of means-tested benefits, several, including the Netherlands and Ireland, have introduced the possibility of splitting payments between partners. Australia has also introduced (as from 1995) a partial individualization of income support for the unemployed, whereby the income test will be applied separately to each partner in a couple and one spouse's earnings will only be counted against the benefit entitlement of the other once the higher earner's income exceeds the cut-off point for entitlement. This was designed primarily as a work incentive measure rather than an explicit move towards independence for women, and its impact has yet to be seen (Saunders, 1995), but in the specific context of social security programmes in Australia it offers an interesting and innovative approach.

The treatment of resources

Turning to the question of the assessment of resources, we find a substantial group of countries that apply, or have the potential to apply, a relatively strict approach. However, they are an interesting and apparently paradoxical combination. Looking at the treatment of earnings, it is first of all the group of Latin and Mediterranean countries, along with Austria and Switzerland, which operate the most stringent tests and allow the least amounts of extra earnings to be retained. In addition there are the Nordic countries of Iceland and Sweden, and in effect Finland, since it is reported that discretionary disregards are not often applied. The same applies to Denmark, even though the guideline earnings disregard is rather higher. Ireland also comes into this group for Supplementary Welfare Allowance, although disregards are available for Unemployment Assistance. The UK also falls into a small group with relatively low disregards, including also Norway, the Netherlands and Japan, though it should be born in mind that in the UK, higher disregards apply to lone parents and that Family Credit in effect provides a tapered earnings disregard. Amongst the countries with higher levels of disregards, which include the antipodean countries and the USA, these vary between client groups and some are available only for a specific period. It is noticeable, however, that Australia and New Zealand, the two countries with entirely selective benefit systems, have means-tests for most of their basic benefits that cut in at a considerably higher level in proportion to benefit rates than do many of those in Europe. This effect is accentuated by the tapered withdrawal rates of benefit, which is unusual outside the English speaking countries.

A similar picture emerges from looking at asset tests. In the group that takes more capital and assets into account can be found first of all Austria and Switzerland, with their highly discretionary and locally-based systems. They are also, as stated above, among those countries that pursue family financial obligations further than most. But this group also includes several of the Scandinavian countries, normally regarded as the most socially liberal. It was among these countries that the principle of family financial obligation appeared weakest in relation to the resource unit for social assistance. Yet in Sweden, for example, it is regarded as reasonable that before having recourse to social assistance people might be expected to sell their house, and also car if they have one, unless there are no public transport alternatives for essential travel. A number of other countries, including the Netherlands, can insist on a home being sold if the value is above prescribed limits, while in Austria and some states of the USA (for General Assistance only), the authorities can take a charge on the equity of a claimant's house to recover benefit if the property is sold.

As regards child maintenance, it is interesting to note that while the controversy over the Child Support Act in the UK has fuelled calls for maintenance to be at least partly disregarded for Income Support, the UK is within the mainstream among the OECD countries in counting it in full against assistance payments. Only the Netherlands and Luxembourg discount it entirely, and Australia and the USA (for Aid to Families with Dependent Children) apply partial disregards. Norway applies a disregard of up to 30 per cent of maintenance received above the minimum guaranteed level for lone parents receiving Transitional Allowance. Child benefit or family allowances are also normally counted in full, unless benefit rates are structured so as not to include child dependency additions.

Conclusion

This chapter has suggested that means-testing as a form of benefit selectivity is growing in importance internationally. The significance of different approaches to the technical and political questions involved is therefore also becoming greater. A comparison of the main social assistance benefits in the developed world suggests some patterns of similarity and difference in approach, which are linked both to social and legal traditions, and to the different roles that assistance schemes play within wider social security systems.

How should we interpret these different patterns? First, it has to be emphasized that looking at means-testing alone provides a somewhat selective view of benefit rules. These elements of the benefit structure cannot be seen in isolation. We need to take into account other important features of the different systems, not least the value of benefits in relation to earnings, in order to see what apparently strict or more generous means-tests actually mean in the context of different countries. It also has to be recognized that the salience of social assistance within the social security systems of different countries is likely to be a factor. Our study found that expenditure on assistance benefits in 1992 varied from less than 1 per cent of the GDP in 10 countries to 3.7 per cent in the USA, 4.7 per cent in the UK, 6.8 per cent in Australia and 13.1 per cent in New Zealand. The percentage of national populations receiving assistance benefits varied in a similar manner. The figures for the latter two countries are of course influenced by their social security systems being almost entirely resource-tested.

Nevertheless, these findings do lead to some interesting speculations. For example, the apparent paradox of finding the toughest means-tests in social-democratic Scandinavia, co-existing with a non-traditional view of family types and obligations, may not be so difficult to explain if we look at the broader social security systems and the role that social assistance plays within them. In all the Nordic countries, receipt of social assistance is seen as, in principle at least, a short-term, last resort measure. Normally, loss of earnings through unemployment or sickness would be dealt with through the social insurance system and the priority is to return to the labour market as soon as possible. Longer-term unemployment and family change may be putting some strain on this model, but at present social assistance recipients are still regarded as needing indi-vidualized, locally-based and discretionary help, only part of which may be in the form of cash. Earnings disregards may simply trap people on benefit and any high replacement rates that may result are seen as largely irrelevant because the work tests and general work ethic, and the stigma attached to receipt of social assistance, should in most cases provide sufficient motivation. In this context, the greater individualization of benefit entitlement, which stems from achievements made in emancipation and opportunities for women throughout society and results in an official view of cohabitation which differs from that in the UK, is not inhibited by considerations of excessive cost.

In a system such as Australia, where virtually all benefits are income and asset-tested (though at varying levels), stigma appears to be much less a factor. Poverty alleviation and the encouragement of work effort then requires a more sophisticated range of instruments, including substantial assets disregards and earned-income 'free areas'. The UK falls somewhere between these two points, and while Income Support itself has only a very limited set of income disregards, it has been necessary to create Family Credit in order to provide incentives within an extensive national means-tested benefit structure.

As regards approaches to the benefit and resources unit, it is perhaps most interesting to note the relative uniformity. With a number of exceptions, where wider family obligations have retained a strong legal foundation, the nuclear family is the norm, in spite of some tentative moves towards forms of individualization. Efforts to shift obligation back on to the wider family seem to be unsuccessful where it has been attempted. Belgian efforts, for example, to oblige local welfare centres to recover benefits from relatives have apparently been difficult to enforce (Lambrechts and Dehaes, 1986). The main examples of countries where these obligations have been preserved in practice are Austria and Switzerland, where the localized and discretionary nature of assistance are key factors. In Switzerland, which is currently being put forward by the UK Government as an exemplar in discussion of possible decentralization of benefits (*Independent*, 9 July 1995), social welfare workers have considerable powers to intervene in, and prescribe for, the lives of assistance recipients (Segalman, 1986) – powers that might seem unacceptably Draconian from a UK perspective. There are examples of unmarried couples being instructed to marry in order to qualify for benefits, while some communes refuse assistance where claimants are judged to be responsible for their circumstances (Borer, 1993). Where receipt of assistance benefits is restricted to small and often marginal groups within a society, and particularly where assessment and delivery of benefits are a matter for local municipalities operating with substantial officer discretion, it is easier to imagine how it might be possible administratively and politically to enforce household and family resource tests beyond the boundaries of the nuclear unit.

In the UK, although increases in non-dependant deductions and extension of the obligations for child maintenance through the Child Support Act could both be argued to have pushed back the boundaries of family financial responsibilities, there have been no general attempts as yet to widen the general definition of family obligations for income maintenance purposes. Where this is happening to some extent is in the care of the elderly, in that relatives are now frequently expected to top-up Income Support payments for older people in residential homes (House of Commons, 1991). It could also be argued that the abolition of Income Support payments for young people aged 16–17 (except in cases of special hardship) has also attempted to redefine family obligations in relation to the benefit system. A move towards a more localized and discretionary system could potentially allow further redefinition of the resource unit, though the experience of other countries suggests that this would be difficult politically, especially in an extensive income support system like that of the UK.

Tony Eardley

Acknowledgment

The author wishes to thank Jonathan Bradshaw, Julia Chilvers, Anne Corden, Keith Hartley and Neil Lunt for their helpful comments.

Notes

1 This chapter is based on part of a comparative study of social assistance schemes commissioned by the Department of Social Security and the Organization for Economic Co-operation and Development (OECD). Any views expressed are, however, those of the author and not necessarily those of either of the commissioning bodies. The full study is published as Eardley *et al.*, 1996 forthcoming.
2 The Department of Social Security tends to prefer the term 'income-related' for benefits such as Income Support, Family Credit and Housing Benefit, but this could be seen as misleading in a comparison with some other systems where income alone is subject to a test and all capital and assets are disregarded.

References

ATKINSON, A. (1992) *The Western Experience with Social Safety Nets*, Welfare State Programme Discussion Paper WSP/80, London: London School of Economics/ Suntory-Toyota International Centre for Economic and Related Disciplines.
ATKINSON, A. (1993) *On Targeting Social Security: Theory and Western Experience with Family Benefits*, Welfare State Programme Discussion Paper WSP/99, London: London School of Economics/Suntory-Toyota International Centre for Economic and Related Disciplines.
BECKERMAN, W. (1979) *Poverty and the Impact of Income Maintenance Programmes in Four Countries*, Geneva: International Labour Office.
BORER, M. (1993) *Das neue Sozialhilfegesetz des Kanton Freiburg von 1991: Probleme der politischen Akzeptanz und ihre Folgen für die Beduftigen*, Freiburg: University of Freiburg, Faculty of Philosophy.
BROWN, J., HAUSMAN, P. and KERGER, A. (1991) *Recommendations on Common Criteria Concerning Sufficient Resources and Social Assistance in the Social Protection Systems*, Luxembourg: CEPS/INSTEAD.
COMMISSION OF THE EUROPEAN COMMUNITIES (1991) *Recommendations on Common Criteria Concerning Sufficient Resources and Social Assistance in the Social Protection Systems*, Draft Recommendation by the Council COM (91)161, 13 May, Brussels.
COMMISSION OF THE EUROPEAN COMMUNITIES (1994) *White Paper – Growth, Competitiveness, Employment: The Challenges and Ways Forward into the 21st Century*, Luxembourg: Office for Official Publications of the European Communities.
DEACON, A. and BRADSHAW, J. (1983) *Reserved for the Poor*, Oxford: Martin Robertson.
EARDLEY, T., BRADSHAW, J., DITCH, J., GOUGH, I. and WHITEFORD, P. (1996, forthcoming) *Social Assistance Schemes in the OECD Countries*, Department of Social

Security Research Report, London: HMSO.

ESAM, P. and BERTHOUD, R. (1991) *Independent Benefits for Men and Women*, London: Policy Studies Institute.

GOUGH, I. (1994) 'Means-testing in the western world', Richard Titmuss Memorial Lecture, Hebrew University of Jerusalem, 31 May.

HOUSE OF COMMONS (1991) *The Financing of Private Residential and Nursing Home Fees*, Fourth Report of the Social Security Committee, Session 1990–1991, London: HMSO.

Independent, (1995) 'Tories plan regional dole rates', 9 July, p. 1.

KIERNAN, K. and ESTAUGH, V. (1993) *Cohabitation: Extra-Marital Childbearing and Social Policy*, London: Family Policy Studies Centre.

LAMBRECHTS, E. and DEHAES, V. (1986) 'Het OCMW en de onderhoudsplicht: en enquete bij 224 Vlaamse OCMWs over kosten en terugvorderingen', Leuven: University of Leuven.

LISTER, R. (1992) *Women's Economic Dependency and Social Security*, EOC Research Discussion Series No. 2, Manchester: Equal Opportunities Commission.

LUNT, N. and CORDEN, A. (1996 forthcoming) *Charging Ahead? Local Authorities' Charging Policies for Community Care*, Social Policy Reports No. 5, York: Social Policy Research Unit.

MILLAR, J. (1994) 'Lone parents and social security policy in the UK', in BALDWIN, S. and FALKINGHAM, J. (Eds) *Social Security and Social Change*, Hemel Hempstead: Harvester Wheatsheaf, pp. 62–75.

MILLAR, J. and WHITEFORD, P. (1993) 'Child support in lone parent families: policies in Australia and the UK', *Policy and Politics*, **21**, 1, pp. 59–72.

MITCHELL, D. (1991) *Welfare States and Welfare Outcomes*, Aldershot: Avebury.

MITCHELL, D., HARDING, A. and GRUEN, F. (1994) 'Targeting welfare', *The Economic Record*, No. 210, September, pp. 315–340.

ORGANISATION FOR ECONOMIC CO-OPERATION AND DEVELOPMENT (1994) *The OECD Jobs Study: Volume 1. Facts, Analysis, Strategies*, Paris: OECD.

ROOM, G. (1990) *'New Poverty' in the EC*, London: Macmillan.

SAUNDERS, P. (1991) 'Selectivity and targeting in income support: the Australian experience', *Journal of Social Policy*, **20**, 3, pp. 299–326.

SAUNDERS, P. (1995) 'Improving work incentives in a means-tested welfare system: the 1994 Australian social security reforms', *Fiscal Studies*, **16**, 2, pp. 47–70.

SEGALMAN, R. (1986) *The Swiss Way of Welfare*, New York: Westport.

WHITEFORD, P. (1994) 'Welfare targeting', *Parliamentary Brief*, **2**, 5, pp. 58–9.

WORLD BANK (1990) *World Development Report 1990*, Oxford: Oxford University Press.

Chapter 6

The Finance of Community Care

Neil Lunt, Russell Mannion and Peter Smith

In April 1993, new arrangements for community care came fully into existence. Local authorities became responsible for assessing the needs of those experiencing difficulties due to ageing, mental illness, learning disabilities or physical disabilities. They were also made responsible for designing a suitable package of care, and for purchasing that package from a range of competing providers. Finance lies at the heart of this public sector activity. In practice there are numerous sources of finance, both explicit and implicit. Conceptually the debate should be widened to understand the interrelationship of finance with eligibility criteria and boundary issues with health services.

A number of other factors have brought the 'financing' of community care sharply into focus: an ageing population structure; declining family networks; desires to curb public spending; and a wealthier population all help to shape discussion. Overlaying these practical issues is a debate surrounding the appropriate levels of state and individual finance, leading into realms of morality, normative judgments and ideology. In brief, paying for care is becoming one of the most pressing policy issues of our time.

The purpose of this chapter is to disentangle some of these issues, to trace existing sources of finance and to show how they are likely to affect the level and quality of the community care programme. As a starting point, a simple model of the demand for and supply of community care is introduced. The various sources of finance are then discussed. The issues covered include: central Government grants to local authorities; the activities of related welfare services, including housing and health; social security benefits; personal sources of finance; and user charges. The chapter concludes by raising some wider issues of discussion.

Background

The origins of community care policy can be traced back some 90 years, when the first provision was made for people with learning disabilities. However, it was not until more recent times that community care was generally adopted as a policy for all vulnerable groups. Arising from a series of well publicized scandals, and a belief that community care may in many cases be a cheaper option than institutional care, there grew throughout the 1960s and 1970s an increasing disenchantment with hospital based care.

However, hospital closures proceeded at a relatively slow pace, and in 1981 the Government decided that the move to community based care should be accelerated (Department of Health and Social Security, 1981). The major stumbling block to community based care was the difficulty of financing the replacement residential care. The financial savings arising from hospital closures accrued to health authorities, whereas local authorities had the responsibility for funding residential care (Wright *et al.*, 1994).

At the same time, reforms to supplementary benefits in 1980 allowed many more people to purchase independent residential and nursing home care. Thus the central Government social security programme became involved in paying for care on a significant scale. What had previously been a discretionary right to means-tested assistance for residential or nursing home fees – used by a minority – was replaced by a clear entitlement to benefit as part of the board and lodgings regulations. There was no parallel entitlement to assist with costs of care in the community. A strong incentive therefore existed for a person who needed care to enter a residential home in the independent sector, even if some sort of domiciliary care may have been more appropriate. Indeed, local authorities had an incentive to encourage such behaviour, as the central Government would bear the costs. The result was an explosion in the number of independent sector homes and of residents in these homes supported by social security. Between 1979 and 1990 the level of Income Support (Supplementary Benefit before April 1988) used for these purposes rose from £10 million per year to £1390 million per year (1993 prices), with the number of claimants increasing from 12000 to 199000 (Darton and Wright, 1993).

A number of reports published in the mid-1980s were severely critical of community care funding and provision. A Health and Social Services Committee (1985) report identified several problems relating to under-resourcing and the lack of co-ordination in the funding and provision of community care services. In the following year a report from the Audit Commission (1986) provided a trenchant critique of perverse incentives and internal policy contradictions, warning of a 'continued waste of resources and, worst still, care and support that is either lacking entirely or inappropriate to the needs of some of the most disadvantaged members of society and the relatives who seek to care for them'.

The concern led directly to the Government commissioning a review by Sir

Roy Griffiths (Griffiths, 1988). Griffiths' term of reference involved an investigation of the use of, rather than the adequacy of, resources. A primary concern of the review was the comparison of the financial arrangements for funding residential and nursing homes with those for domiciliary care. Most of Griffiths' recommendations were accepted by the central Government and were incorporated into the White Paper *Caring for People* (Department of Health, 1989) and the subsequent National Health Service and Community Care Act (1990).

Underpinning the legislation were six key objectives for service delivery:

1   promoting the development of domiciliary, day and respite services to enable people to live in their own homes wherever feasible and sensible;
2   ensuring that service providers make practical support for carers a high priority;
3   making prior assessment of need and good case management the cornerstone of good quality care;
4   promoting the development of a flourishing independent sector alongside good quality public services;
5   clarifying the responsibilities of agencies, so making it easier to hold them to account for their performance;
6   securing better value for taxpayers' money by introducing a new funding structure for community care.

Under the new arrangements, local authority social service departments have been designated the lead agency for developing community care. They have been given responsibility, in collaboration with health and housing authorities, for making assessments of the care needs of individuals. Having identified an individual's needs, they must design a package of care, within local budget constraints, and purchase that care from a choice of providers in the public, private and voluntary sectors. Packages of care are now organized by 'care managers', many of whom have control over devolved budgets for purchasing care. The reforms therefore introduce a quasi-market into community care, along the lines of those already in place in schools and health care (LeGrand and Bartlett, 1993). Underlying the reforms is a presumption that the disciplines of the market will encourage those providing care (whether independent or public sector) to be more efficient in running their services (Lunt *et al.*, 1994).

A Model of Demand for, and Supply of, Community Care

An important point to recognize is that, within any local authority, the funds directly available for community care are cash-limited. This being the case, some rationing device is required to ensure that cash limits are adhered to. Local

Key Financing Issues in Community Care

The model (Figure 6.1) in the discussion shall be returned to. However, this section considers the more important financing factors affecting the supply and demand curves. Local authority budgets and community care finance, and health and housing are the supply factors considered. The demand factors considered are the range of personal finances, and the section incorporates the issue of user charges, which may affect both demand and supply.

Local authority budgets and the Revenue Support Grant

The primary direct sources for finance of community care are the funds made available for the programme by a local authority. Local authority budgeting decision-making processes are complex, and defy easy analysis (Elcock and Jordan, 1987). However, two factors have a profound impact on almost all local authority budgets. The first is the level of general Revenue Support Grant provided by central Government. Broadly speaking, all expenditure in excess of this grant must be met from the local Council Tax. The second, even more important influence, is the expenditure 'cap' set by central Government. Most local authorities with social service responsibilities spend at this cap, so it effectively determines the aggregate local authority budget. The local authority budgeting process is therefore in practice principally concerned with the allocation of an externally determined sum between services. Within this framework, the community care budget will reflect local preferences *vis à vis* other services such as transportation and education.

The Revenue Support Grant (RSG) is designed to enable a local authority to charge a standard level of local taxation if it delivers some standard level of service to its residents. Central to the calculation of the RSG is the local authority's Standard Spending Assessment (SSA). This is central Government's estimate of the local costs of delivering a standard level of services, given the area's social and economic circumstances. SSAs are developed for individual services using a variety of statistical methods. They are then aggregated to yield an authority's total SSA, which forms the basis for the RSG calculation. The SSA has also become the central Government's basis for setting a local authority's budget cap (Society of County Treasurers, 1994).

In 1994/5 the personal social services SSA had four components: children; older people (residential); older people (domiciliary); and other social services. In itself, the personal social services SSA is not in principle intended directly to influence the local personal social services budget. Indeed, because their budgets are built-up on a different basis to SSAs, many local authorities find it difficult to compare their spending on particular services with the associated SSA (Audit Commission, 1993). However, the personal social services SSA does in practice have a particularly important impact on the community care budget, because in 1994/5 it formed the basis for the authority's Special Transitional Grant, discussed in the next section.

Central Government Special Transitional Grant

The Special Transitional Grant (STG) provided by the central Government is a further input into community care financing. The grant can only be spent on community care services for new referrals in the budgeting year, and 85 per cent must be spent on private or voluntary sector providers. The conditional nature of the STG has the effect of 'ring-fencing' spending on new referrals, ensuring that the STG is spent on community care, and not diverted to other budgets, as can occur with the RSG. Existing community care commitments (that is, those inherited from the previous year) are not ring-fenced in this way. An area's STG reflects the Government's estimate of how much it should spend on new users of community care, taking account of local demographic and socio-economic circumstances. Traditionally, local authority budgets are set, net of user charges, so that the community care budget will reflect the expected income from user charges, to be discussed in more detail below.

As mentioned, the STG is determined on the basis of an area's SSA. In 1994/5 an area's STG was constructed so that 75 per cent of it was based on the older persons residential component, 10 per cent on the older persons domiciliary component, and 15 per cent on the 'other adult services' component. The total STG for England was £736 million (Association of County Councils, 1994). Over time, it is to be expected that the weighting on the residential sector will decrease relative to that on the domiciliary sector, as the intended shift from institutional to community care takes place.

The health sector

Outside the local authority sector, the most important public sector services are those provided by the National Health Service. These have two broad components: hospital and community services; and primary care. In the hospital sector, there is a small volume of joint finance between health authorities and local authorities, which may have some bearing on community care. Of much greater significance, however, are the policies that a health authority has towards the discharge of the long-term ill into the community. At one extreme, a hard line health authority might insist that its providers discharge all patients into the community at the earliest possible opportunity, placing much of the burden of after-care immediately onto the community care programme. However, in areas where there is a better relationship with local authorities, it may be that the health authority is prepared to shoulder more of the financial burden of social care, thereby implicitly relieving some of the pressure on local community care. A complicating factor in the hospital sector is the increasing importance of general practice fundholding, whereby some of the health authority is devolved to general practitioners, who purchase a wide range of procedures under contracts that are independent from those of the health authority.

The central Government has released guidelines on the limits of NHS responsibility for continuing care (Department of Health, 1995), which emphasize the need for clear agreements covering the respective responsibilities of health and local authorities. However, the document leaves the precise definition of continuing care open to local interpretation. It nevertheless seeks to circumscribe the responsibilities of the NHS for continuing care in circumstances where the patient is in need of regular, complex or unpredictable clinical care, or a period of rehabilitation. If the patient does not fall within these criteria, and refuses to be discharged into a nursing or residential home, the health authority is entitled to charge the local authority for the social care element of the patient's package. A key consideration in this context, is that, while NHS patients are not charged for their care, community care users may be liable for charges, usually subject to a means-test.

In the primary care sector, the principal providers are general practitioners, who – although nominally administered by Family Health Service Authorities – have traditionally enjoyed considerable autonomy. Again, substantial latitude exists in the interpretation of what constitutes health care and what constitutes social care, so the attitudes of general practitioners will be influential on the demand for community care. There have traditionally been few formal links between local authorities and the primary care sector. However, proposed merging of Health Authorities and Family Health Service Authorities may offer the opportunity for a more useful dialogue.

The housing sector

The state of the local housing stock can have a profound impact on the demand for community care, particularly in relation to physically disabled persons and the provision of sheltered accommodation. For example, relatively trivial adaptations to a person's house, such as the provision of wheelchair access, can considerably enhance independence and reduce the need for assistance. The finance of housing is a complex area involving a wide range of agencies, and co-ordination with social service departments may therefore be difficult.

Local Government housing departments are responsible for managing local authority housing stock, and for administering grants for the adaptation and improvement of private housing stock. The local authority housing sector is financed principally through revenue from rental income. Relatively minor adaptations for disabled people can be financed directly from within that fund. Major developments are considered capital expenditure. The provision of new local authority housing stock is severely constrained by central Government limits on capital expenditure. A local authority's capital plans are set out in its Housing Investment Programme (HIP), which is a bid to the central Government for a capital allocation of housing. In the light of these bids, the Government makes an annual capital allocation to every authority, of which 40 per cent is based on a complex 'Generalized Needs Index' formula, and 60 per cent on discretion. A small part of the allocation is based on assessed needs for disabled and elderly users.

Thus, in securing suitable accommodation for potential users of community care, close liaison between housing and social service departments will be necessary, in relation to both revenue and capital expenditure. Outside London and the metropolitan areas, such co-operation is complicated by the fact that community care is administered by counties, while housing is a responsibility of lower level district councils. Similar considerations also apply to the link with housing associations. The activities of the associations are supervised by the Housing Corporation, which provides capital and revenue grants in the form of Housing Association Grants (capital) and Revenue Deficit Grants (revenue). The allocation of these grants is determined on the basis of bids by individual housing associations. Clearly the responsiveness of local housing associations to community care issues may have a significant impact on user needs.

In the private housing sector, various renovation grants are financed by the central Government, and administered by local Government. Of most direct relevance to community care is the Disabled Facilities Grant, which the authority must provide if the relevant works are 'necessary and appropriate to meet the needs of the disabled occupant', and are reasonable and practicable to carry out (Bucknall, 1991, p. 261). To that end, the housing department must consult the relevant social services department. The principal adaptations covered by the grant relate to access to the accommodation, movement around the accommodation, and improvements to heating and cooking facilities. The local authority may pay a discretionary grant if the required adaptations do not fall under the terms of the Disabled Facilities Grant. The grant is means-tested, and 60 per cent of it is reimbursed directly by the central Government.

At the time of writing, the system of renovation grants is under review as the Government seeks to restrain expenditure in this area. The likely outcome is less direct central Government support and more local discretion in the allocation of grants. In respect of community care, such developments would make close liaison between social services and housing departments even more important.

Personal finance

Discussion so far has outlined what may be considered to be collective forms of finance (financed through the local or national tax systems). The finance is distributed either top-down from central Government to local authorities direct, or flows into community care provision through health authorities, or takes the form of revenue raised direct by local authorities. Decisions have to be made at the local level on how to allocate this funding.

There are, however, a further range of personal sources of finance that have both direct and indirect implications for the community care programme. Of central importance are the resources commanded by individual users or potential users. In this respect, it should be noted that an individual's assessed *need* for community care depends not only on their physical capabilities, but also on the support received from friends and family, and from the characteristics of the physical environment. Indeed as Griffiths (1988) noted:

> The proposals take as their starting point that . . . the first task of publicly provided services is to support and where possible strengthen [these] networks of carers.

Thus, for example, relatively modest physical incapacity may necessitate significant community care resources if the user's social (or physical environment) is unsuitable (Phillipson and Walker, 1986; Oliver, 1990).

Charging or paying

Prior to the discussion of determinants for personal finance, mention is necessary of the alternative ways that this finance can be drawn into the system. The ways of utilizing personal finance is two fold: by the individual paying directly; or through a local authority's charging policy 'syphoning' private resources. In spite of frequent discussions surrounding dependency, frail older people care for themselves most of the time (Wilson, 1993), and most of those requiring assistance also design their own care packages (Wilson, 1994): including domestic help; gardening; personal care; and transport. Furthermore, informal care has traditionally underpinned much of the formal social care sector.

Local authorities are empowered to charge for care services, both residential and nursing accommodation and domiciliary provision. Central Government in its annual settlement with local authorities is making the explicit assumption that users should be charged for community care services (Department of the Environment, 1995). While charges for residential and nursing care are subject to national statute, authorities have greater discretion when charging for domiciliary services. Consequently a plethora of domiciliary charging policies has developed locally, making different assumptions about income, savings, capital and benefits and their use in paying for care. A charging policy, for example, may offer a free service to those receiving Income Support; require a contribution from those receiving either Attendance Allowance or Disability Living Allowance; and require those with savings over a certain level to pay the full cost of their service.

Clearly an individual's financial resources will have an impact on demand for community care. At one extreme – depending on the local authority's charging policies – a wealthy individual may have nothing to gain from using the community care programme, and may instead opt for a private care contract. In practice, those living in middle class areas are more likely to buy a greater range of care services for themselves (Wilson, 1994). At the other extreme, a low income individual may qualify for care and be subject to no charges, in which case the community care programme bears the entire cost.

Personal sources of finance principally comprise occupational pensions, savings, earnings and capital assets. A combination of demographic and ideological factors, combined with the belief that many individuals have access to rising income and wealth, has prompted a view that (where possible) individuals should contribute to the costs of their own care out of their own resources. This is seen particularly in relation to older people who consume the greatest amount of community care resources. According to this view, through suitable life-cycle planning, citizens should accumulate assets or insurance over their early lives, and use the proceeds to pay for community care towards the end of their lives.

The evidence takes a less optimistic view. Walker (1988) is very sceptical about the elderly being able to pay their own way. He notes, that any increases in income are from a low base and that furthermore, pensioners are not a homogenous group. Perhaps 1 in 10 could contribute to costs of their care without going into poverty, while those with greatest incapacity are most likely to have the least financial resources. More recent evidence would seem to support this. For example, Hancock and Weir (1994) warn of the dangers of considering pensioners as a homogenous group.

Determinants of personal finance

For the majority of community care services users, access to alternative forms of funds, in order to pay for care would seem limited. Rising coverage of occupational pensions has been suggested, as a source of finance to pay for care. Coverage is, however, uneven: Gibbs (1991) notes that access to schemes, favours men rather than women. Moreover, the real value of these schemes often declines year after year, as many are not indexed to inflation. In addition, personal pensions are unlikely to have any real financial benefit for many of those retiring before 2020 (Craig, 1992). Finally, much of the real value of personal pensions is lost to the individual because of the removal of entitlement to means-tested benefits (Walker *et al.*, 1989). The situation is accentuated, because the majority of people over pensionable age have little or no money from personal earnings and this trend is increasing (Guillemard, 1989) whilst the majority of older people have little savings income that could be utilised for care (Gibbs, 1991). Older council tenants and older housing association tenants, would seem particularly disadvantaged in this respect (Maclennan *et al.* 1990).

Some commentators have outlined the importance of wealth in the debate (Gibbs and Oldman, 1993). The principal asset available for many older people is the family home – 50 per cent of the population over 65 are home owners. A crucial issue in relation to the self-financing of community care is, therefore, the extent to which housing equity is considered a legitimate source of financing. Clearly, in principle, home owners can release the equity; either by selling their homes or by using a variety of equity release instruments. However, despite the proliferation of such schemes, a number of studies (Gibbs, 1991; Oldman, 1991) indicate that there would, in many cases, still be considerable gaps between money realized through equity release schemes, and money required to pay for long term care. Gibbs and Oldman (1993) conclude that only about one in 10 older people possess high equity and high income.

Another possible method of paying for community care is to use private insurance. Again, a number of studies have indicated that private insurance will only be a realistic option for a small proportion of community care users. Studies by Oldman (1991) and Henwood (1990) have shown that the majority of older people are unlikely to be able to finance their own care through private insurance.

Social security benefits

One of the most important sources of personal finance available to fund community care is the range of social security benefits. The Department of Social Security continues to be *directly* involved in financing community care for those who were residents of nursing or residential homes, and in receipt of the higher levels of income support before April 1993. These residents have what are known as 'preserved rights'.

Of greater interest, however, are those social security benefits that may be *indirectly* utilized to construct a private package of care, or alternatively, taken by the local authority as a contribution towards an assessed package of care. In macro terms, total benefit expenditure paid in 1993/4 to older people (£36 763 million) and disabled people (£18 377 million) is considerable. A variety of different benefits flow through the social security system into community care. For some monies the relationship with community care is relatively clear, while for others the relationship is less transparent. Key sources are highlighted here.

Means-tested benefits

Income Support is the major form of income maintenance in the social security system. It operates in conjunction with a range of premiums: disability premium; severe disability premium; disabled child premium; higher pensioner premium and carers' premium. Many local authorities consider some of these benefits as chargeable income: severe disability premium (an extra amount of benefit to severely disabled people living on their own and most likely to need extra support and care) is an example of this. This understanding is, however, contested.

The second major type of means-tested benefits for more direct use of community care, are those of Community Care Grants. These grants are a discretionary part of the Social Fund arrangements, and decisions are taken by Social Fund Officers within a fixed framework of directions and a more flexible framework of guidance. The Grants are 'mainly intended to help certain vulnerable people in receipt of Income Support to re-establish themselves following a period of residential and institutional care'. They are also intended to prevent people moving into inappropriate institutional care. In 1993/4 there were 1 244 000 applications, and 26 per cent were awarded one-off grants averaging £288 each.

Non means-tested benefits

Attendance Allowance is a benefit that is payable to a person (over 65) who is severely disabled, physically or mentally, enough that he or she requires, from another person, 'frequent attention' or 'continual supervision' during the day, and 'prolonged or repeated attention' or 'continual supervision' at night. It is payable at two levels. The Disability Living Allowance (DLA) was introduced in 1992, with care and mobility components, to complement Attendance Allowance. The DLA (care component) is for those under 65 who would have previously applied for Attendance Allowance, and is paid at one of three levels. Whilst the DLA (mobility component) replaced mobility allowance, for those 'unable to walk' or 'virtually unable to walk' and is paid at one of two levels. Neither Attendance Allowance nor DLA is means-tested or contributory.

Invalid Care Allowance (ICA) is a benefit for carers, of working age, who regularly spend 35 hours a week caring for a severely disabled person. It is another form of indirect community care funding. For a carer to claim, the disabled person must themselves be in receipt of either the highest or middle rate of DLA (care); Attendance Allowance; or Constant Attendance Allowance.

Invalidity Benefit and Severe Disablement Allowance are the main replacement benefits for those disabled people unable to work. Invalidity Benefit is intended for those who have made the necessary contributions, while Severe Disablement Allowance is for those who have not. There exists a range of other benefits, including Disability Working Allowance, war pensions and allowances, and Industrial Injuries Disablement Benefits. The above examples are intended merely to give a flavour of the range of benefits that may flow into the funding of community care.

An important consideration is that the purpose of benefits is rarely articulated, and purposes can be 'essentially contested'. As Berthoud and Horton (1990) note, for example, a common assumption is that Attendance Allowance was designed as a payment towards the cost of care. It can, however, be spent on anything and may well be subsumed into the general household budgeting process. Questions relating to the internal distribution of resources (labour and money) within, and between, families have until recently been relatively unexplored.

Conclusion

This chapter has identified the principal sources of finance for community care in the United Kingdom, and the sources we have discussed relate to health authorities; local authorities; the Department of Social Security; and personal sources of household income (earnings, pensions, insurance, savings and personal equity).

Continuing health care in the community is principally provided by the National Health Service. It is directly funded from central taxation – with most services delivered free at the point of use. The general practitioner service, funded by Family Health Service Authorities, is also becoming an increasingly important source of support for people with continuing care needs in the community. In addition, local authorities purchase and provide a range of personal social services, funded by a combination of central and local taxation, and increasingly by user charges.

Health and social services, however, support only a small fraction of the personal care needs of dependent people in the community. According to the Office of Population, Censuses and Surveys (OPCS) survey of disability (Martin *et al.*, 1988) only 14 per cent of adults receive help of any kind from organized services. The overwhelming majority of personal care is undertaken within, and by the community, often within the family – usually by a partner, or adult sons or daughters. The care of older people is still seen as a private domain and a family responsibility. Social security benefits represent the main statutory financial support for dependent people and their carers.

Taken together, these alternative funding channels represent a complex network of finance for community care: funded from collective and personal resources. Clearly such a complex system of finance can have both advantages and disadvantages. On the positive side, such a multiplicity of funding sources can, perhaps, offer the possibility of flexibility and innovation in the construction of individual care arrangements. Conversely, it is susceptible to failure in securing comprehensive coverage, leaving gaps and inequities in service provision. To avoid this, it is necessary for health and social services, along with the Department of Social Security, to work together to encourage a seamless service of health and social care needs.

Superimposed on this complex system of financing is the fundamental economic problem of resource scarcity in the face of apparently insatiable need. Within the constraints of finite resources, the various funding bodies we have outlined must ration care. We have used a simple economic (demand and supply) model to examine the impact of changing various aspects of the system of finance on the delivery of community care services, and the eligibility criteria by which they are rationed. The important point to note, is that changes in one aspect of community care finance can have (often unintended) repercussions in other sectors of provision. For instance, any reduction in the levels of social security support for carers could result in some people withdrawing from their caring role: leading to local authority social services departments having to provide more domiciliary services, or even fund a residential placement. Policy in this area must, therefore, consider the 'displacement effects' that can result from changes in the funding base. The supply and demand model suggests that two important effects are likely to be the numbers of people admitted to the community care programme, and the eligibility criteria.

To conclude, three key issues surrounding the future nature of community care finance are identified. First, there is the problem of deciding on the correct balance of collective and personal finance for community care. The central thrust of recent policy (for example, the extension of charges) has been to shift more of the costs of provision on to users and their families. Such a policy can help reduce public expenditure, and reduce the national and local tax burden. The personal cost to some families, however, may be high and in extreme cases may result in users withdrawing from services. Increased use of means-testing to target resources may have dysfunctional consequences. For example, it may introduce a poverty trap, and discourage people from retaining their own resources to pay for care. It may promote stigma among users. And it may also produce a two tier system of care, comprising those wealthy enough to fund their own care arrangements, and the remainder of the population relying on a poorly funded residualized public service. Achieving the right balance between collective and personal finance for community care is one of the thorniest problems ahead.

A second important issue to be addressed by national and local Government is deciding on the extent to which the finance for community care services is devolved to users. In particular, should direct payments be made to those entitled to support from the community care programme? These payments would enable users to make their own arrangements for personal and domestic assistance. It would transfer the role of purchasing and monitoring care to the individual, and limit the role of the local authority to needs assessor and financier.

Disability groups have argued strongly for the extension of direct payment schemes as, in theory at least, such arrangements can give service users increased choice and control over the range and type of services they receive. However, direct payment schemes could also have drawbacks because they are of relevance principally in circumstances where users are able to manage their money effectively. This does not apply to many older people, people with learning disabilities and those suffering from mental illness. A further potential drawback of direct payments is that this cash can be used to purchase items that are unrelated to community care. For instance, additional cash in the form of a direct payment could be used to pay a fuel bill or other household contingencies. The choice in this context may effectively be one of preventing a fuel disconnection, or paying for a home help. Therefore, a necessary tension exists between targeting and controlling community care finance in terms of social welfare (seen as a merit good) and individual choice and control. One possible solution to this problem is to provide finance in an intermediate form such as a voucher, so offering choice to users, while ensuring money is spent on community care services.

The third key issue relates to the level of resources to be devoted to community care. In a system which relies heavily on collective (state) funding, this is clearly a direct concern of policy makers. However, even in a system funded predominantly from private sources, there are innumerable collective policy actions, such as tax relief, that may affect the resources allocated to community care.

In order to summarize the issues, Figure 6.2 characterizes community care finance in two dimensions, relating respectively to the *raising* of finance, and to the *spending* of community care funds. Here, the simplifying assumption is made that finance can be raised and spent, either collectively or individually. In box 1 the situation is such as in the National Health Service where finance is predominantly both raised and spent centrally. In box 2 is the situation that local authority charges give rise to, where finance is raised from individual resources

		RAISING FUNDS	
		Collective	**Individual**
SPENDING FUNDS	**Collective**	1 'Monolithic' state supply	2 User charges
	Individual	3 Direct payments, vouchers	4 Private care

Figure 6.2: Alternative approaches to the financing of community care

but spent collectively. Box 3 represents a situation of direct payments or vouchers, where finance is raised centrally, but where users themselves purchase care. Box 4 represents a free market situation, where individuals purchase care (or care insurance) using their own resources. In the United Kingdom, formal finance for community care is predominantly reflected by box 1, however we are seeing a shift towards box 2, as user charges are increasingly used to finance care, and towards boxes 3 and 4, as direct payment schemes attract more interest.

It is useful to locate the UK financing system for community care within a cross-national context. Esping-Anderson (1990) has suggested that welfare states cluster into three distinct regime-types: liberal, corporatist, and social democratic. These regime-types can also be used to model national financing systems.

Liberal welfare state regimes are characterized by modest social insurance coverage, and a limited amount of means-testing. There is statutory support for health and social services, which are largely targeted at the poor. The market is the principal allocator of welfare resources, the state only provides a residual minimum and sometimes subsidizes private welfare schemes. The low level of state services in liberal welfare state regimes means that personal resources, family and charity play a major role in the provision of services. Finance for community care services is derived predominantly from personal resources. This relates to box 4 of Figure 6.2.

In corporatist welfare states, state finance is predominant with the market having only a marginal role to play in the financing and allocation of community care services. Despite this, the welfare regimes are essentially conservative in nature with little overt income redistribution, and the state supports the maintenance of status and class differentials. Few services are provided to support the family, and the state only intervenes where family care breaks down.

Social democratic welfare regimes have a financing system the objective of which is to promote equality and develop high standards of care. Usually the whole population is covered by a comprehensive insurance programme, although this may be graduated. The market has very little role to play, and there is little private insurance for long-term care. In this model, the state bears the primary responsibility for the care of dependent people. This is reflected in box 1.

The UK system of finance does not fit easily into any of the three models – indeed it could be said to contain elements of all three. For instance, the financing of the NHS mirrors closely the social democratic model. On the other hand, the social security system, with its emphasis on means-testing, is gradually becoming more residualized. The family and informal carers continue to be the main providers and site of care-giving. Until some consensus is reached on the issues raised here, community care is likely to continue to be one of the most keenly debated aspects of public policy.

Acknowledgment

Part of this work was funded by the Economic and Social Research Council (ESRC) Local Governance Initiative project L311253059, 'Targeting and Control in the Finance of Local Governance'.

References

ASSOCIATION OF COUNTY COUNCILS (1994) *Revenue Support Grant: England, 1994/1995*, London: ACC.

AUDIT COMMISSION (1986) *Making a Reality of Community Care*, London: HMSO.

AUDIT COMMISSION (1993) *Passing the Bucks: The Impact of SSAs on Economy, Efficiency and Effectiveness*, London: HMSO.

BERTHOUD, R. and HORTON, C. (1990) *The Attendance Allowance and the Costs of Caring*, London: Policy Studies Institute.

BUCKNALL, B. (1991) *Housing Finance*, 2nd Edn, London: Chartered Institute of Public Finance and Accountance.

CRAIG, G. (1992) *Cash or Care: A Question of Choice?* York: Social Policy Research Unit, University of York.

DARTON, R.A. and WRIGHT, K.G. (1993) 'Changes in the provision of long-stay care 1970–1990', *Health & Social Care in the Community*, **1**(2), pp. 11–25.

DEPARTMENT OF THE ENVIRONMENT (1995) *Standard Spending Assessments: Guide to Methodology*, London: DOE.

DEPARTMENT OF HEALTH (1989) *Caring for People: Community Care in the Next Decade and Beyond*, Cm 849, London: HMSO.

DEPARTMENT OF HEALTH (1995) *Guidance on Continuing Care Responsibilities*, London: DH.

DEPARTMENT OF HEALTH AND SOCIAL SECURITY (1981) *Growing Older*, Cmnd 8173, London: HMSO.

ELCOCK, H. and JORDON, G. (Eds) (1987) *Learning from Local Authority Budgeting*, Aldershot: Avebury.

ESPING-ANDERSON, G. (1990) *The Three Worlds of Welfare Capitalism*, Cambridge: Polity.

GIBBS, I. (1991) 'Income, capital and the cost of care in old age', *Ageing and Society*, **11**(4), pp. 373–97.

GIBBS, I. and OLDMAN, C. (1993) *Housing Wealth in Later Life: A Mixed Blessing*, York: Centre for Housing Policy, University of York.

GRIFFITHS, R. (1988) *Community Care: Agenda for Action*, London: HMSO.

GUILLEMARD, A.M. (1989) 'The trend towards early labour force withdrawal', in JOHNSON, P., CONRAD, C. and THOMSON, D. (Eds) *Workers vs Pensioners*, Manchester: University Press.

HANCOCK, R. and WEIR, P. (1994) 'The financial well-being of elderly people', *Social Policy Research Findings*, **57**, York: Joseph Rowntree Foundation.

HENWOOD, M. (1990) 'Long-term care insurance: Has it a future?', HARRISON, A. (Ed.) *Health Care UK*, pp. 97–105, London: Kings Fund.

HOUSE OF COMMONS (1985) *Second Report from the Social Services Committee*, 1984/5, Community Care, London: HMSO.

LEGRAND, J. and BARTLETT, W. (1993) *Quasi-markets and Social Policy*, London: Macmillan.

LUNT, N., MANNION, R. and SMITH, P. (1994) 'Theories of the market: the case of community care', paper presented to IFS Seminar on Local Government Finance, London, November.

MACLENNAN, D., GIBB, K. and MORE, A. (1990) *Paying for Britain's Housing*, York: Joseph Rowntree Foundation.

MARTIN, L,. MELTZER, H. and ELLIOT, D. (1988) *The Prevalence of Disability Among Adults*, London: HMSO.

National Health Service and Community Care Act (1990), London: HMSO.

OLDMAN, C. (1991) *Paying for Care: Personal Sources of Funding Care*, York: Joseph Rowntree Foundation.

OLIVER, M. (1990) *The Politics of Disablement*, London: Macmillan.

PHILLIPSON, C. and WALKER, A. (Eds) (1986) *Ageing and Social Policy: A Critical Assessment*, Aldershot: Gower.

SOCIETY OF COUNTY TREASURERS (1994) *Standard Spending Indicators 1994/1995*, Maidstone: SCT.

WALKER, R. (1988) 'The financial resources of the elderly; paying your own way in old age', in BALDWIN, S., PARKER, G. and WALKER, R. (Eds) *Social Security and Community Care*, Aldershot: Avebury.

WALKER, R., HARDMAN, G. and HUTTON, S. (1989) 'The occupational pension trap', *Journal of Social Policy*, **18**(4), pp. 575–93.

WILSON, G. (1993) 'Conflicts in case management', *Social Policy and Administration*, **27**, pp. 109–123.

WILSON, G. (1994) 'Assembling their own care packages: payments for care by men and women in advanced old age', *Health & Social Care in the Community*, **2**, pp. 283–91.

WRIGHT, K.G., HAYCOX, A. and LEEDHAM, I. (1994) *Evaluating Community Care: Services for People with Learning Disabilities*, Buckingham: Open University Press.

Chapter 7

Community Care: Some Reflections on an Ideal

John Horton

This chapter on community care is intended as a companion piece to the preceding chapter rather than a direct commentary on it. Moreover, I approach the topic as someone who is not an expert on social policy or welfare economics. Instead, the aim is to step back from some of the technical details of policy and implementation, and to look in a very general way at what the idea of community care could mean; what values inform it; why it might be a worthwhile ideal to pursue; and to what problems it gives rise.

Background

It is helpful to begin, however, by briefly explaining a couple of the more important considerations that lie behind this enquiry. First, there is the almost uniformly hostile press that current community care policy, based on the 1990 Act, and implemented since 1993, has received. It is not that much of the criticism of Government policy is unjustified, motivated as the policy mostly has been by narrow ideological dogma and the desire of the Treasury to cut public expenditure, particularly on welfare provision, it is not surprising that there have been predictable and serious difficulties with the implementation of it. Rather, what has been interesting, and perhaps surprising, is the apparent hostility (most forcefully expressed by those on the political left) to aspects of the policy which, if implemented in a less doctrinaire and more financially generous spirit, one might expect to be widely welcomed – not least by those on the political left. What has been particularly alarming about the general hostility is the prominence of law and order, or 'disciplinary' concerns. Many of the sensationalized stories in the popular press have been about the dangers to others of releasing people from institutions into the community, unintentionally showing that the real worry is frequently less about caring for such people than about controlling them.

The second consideration motivating this enquiry arises from a degree of scepticism about the necessity and desirability of the widespread and continuing trend towards the professionalization of the provision for all forms of welfare, including the kinds of social care with which this paper is mostly concerned. One can question the cult of expertise, and the appropriateness of specialist provision, to which institutionalization has often been concomitant, while acknowledging the obvious truths that there is an important role for professionals, that there are significant areas of expert knowledge and that institutionalization is sometimes undeniably preferable to any alternative. No part of the ensuing argument supports, or depends upon, any thoroughgoing libertarianism, of either left or right-wing stripes. What is of concern is the way in which the very idea of 'caring' has become transformed into a highly specialized activity, entirely the province of properly trained professionals, and all that is required of non-experts is the money to enable the experts to deliver their service. This is an understanding of care that we ought to be less willing to embrace.

The Meaning of Community Care

One difficulty in considering community care is its vagueness, and the way in which it has been used to mean quite different things (Bulmer, 1987; Parker, 1990). Inevitably, this is a source of frustration to social scientists and policy analysts who like to work with determinate and operationalizable concepts in order to develop and test empirical hypotheses; though it is a situation with which moral and political philosophers feel more comfortable. Social scientists are inclined to be impatient with what they perceive as vague aspirations and ideals; but vagueness is not the same as emptiness and, as Aristotle long ago remarked, we should not expect more precision than a subject allows.

Numerous chapters in this volume rightly stress the importance of objective empirical research in assessing the effects of particular policies, especially their unintended consequences. However, such empirical research, no matter how well-devised and conducted, cannot answer all our questions about social policies. Any social policy will be informed by some values, as chapters in this volume acknowledge. Such policies exist to give effect to those values and it is impossible to make any overall judgement of a policy without some engagement with those values. Of course, for some purposes we can assume certain goals and focus exclusively on the effectiveness of various means to achieve them. But this *is* to ignore a crucial component of any overall evaluation, in which goals too need to be discussed and assessed. Moreover, with respect to many policies it is impossible to make a sharp distinction between means and ends. What is being attempted is inextricably intertwined with how it is being undertaken. The consideration of values, therefore, is not something that can be set aside in assessing social policy, not something that is mere frippery or light relief from the serious business of empirical investigation; even though it introduces a complicating element that is not amenable to treatment by the methods of social science, and raises issues which are not resolvable by empirical enquiry.

It is clear that while there is much disagreement about the meaning of community care there are also some relatively fixed points on which there is considerable consensus. For example, at the heart of community care policies lies the move away from care in specialized residential institutions to home-based care (Department of Health, 1989; Challis and Hugman, 1993). One might express this by saying that the aim is to provide care *in* the community, in the sense of enabling those being cared for to lead as 'normal' a life as possible, rather than taking them outside of that life. No doubt this formulation is far too simple, but the broad idea, at least, does not seem too difficult to grasp. Nor does it seem hard to see why such a shift, to the extent that it is feasible, should be thought desirable. Avoiding unnecessarily dislocating people's lives; encouraging or facilitating their autonomy; increasing the scope for choice and self-determination; supporting a sense that they are full members of society – all seem to be uncontroversially valuable. Inevitably, some forms of care cannot be home-based and others may be prohibitively expensive, so community care will not always be feasible. The point, however, is that, generally speaking, institutionalization is not in itself a good thing and that when it can reasonably be avoided, it should be.

No doubt there are important and interesting ethical issues which arise specifically from this aspect of community care. For example, there are difficult questions about the legitimate scope for paternalistic intervention and acceptable levels of risk but they will not be the concern of this chapter. Rather, the focus will be on a more controversial and obscure thought, which is also sometimes associated with the idea of community care, namely that the care should be provided not only *in* the community but, in a distinctive sense, *by* the community. Here, our attention is directed towards who provides the care. This idea needs further elaboration. In particular there is an ambiguity in the phrase 'those who provide the care', which might mean simply those who pay for the care, or alternatively it might mean those who undertake the activities that comprise the caring. It is the latter sense which is crucial to this conception of community care.

Of course funding cannot be ignored and it is important to remember, as Lunt *et al.* (in Chapter 6) point out, that the 'costs' of the care need not all be borne by those undertaking the caring. They discuss several forms of financing, some of which will impose less financial burdens on the carers than others, though it is always likely to be the case that some costs, particularly time, will not be fully compensated (Twigg and Atkin, 1994). So 'community care' in the sense in which it is used here, does not have any very precise implications about how care is to be funded, although it is certainly true that any adequate and equitable community care policy will need substantial support (both financial and material) from Government. Equally, there is likely to be the need for some economically unrequited commitment on the part of carers, or their families. This ideal of community care necessarily relies on the existence of certain beneficent motivations if it is to be practically effective, and it is a mistake to think that these can or should entirely be eliminated by any 'fair' system of welfare provision.

Thus, what is central to this ideal of community care is that more of the caring (that is the practical activities of caring) should be the responsibility of non-specialists or non-professionals; very roughly, this means people whose career or paid employment is not to provide such care. Kin, friends, neighbours, colleagues and members of voluntary associations are examples of these non-professional providers of care. Spelling out the idea in this way helps to avoid some of the difficulties in attempting to answer the question of what is meant by the 'community' in community care; though this thorny issue is not one that can be entirely circumvented, and we shall need to return to it towards the end of the chapter. It is this sense of the ideal of community care that is to be looked at a little more closely.

Care as a Specialist Service

To begin with, it might be illuminating to set against the ideal of community care an alternative picture of the provision of care. On this account, care is a service, intended to meet authoritatively defined needs, and the aim should be to provide it as efficiently and effectively as possible. This is best done through specialist organizations and professionals who have the requisite expertise. The point of care is to objectively improve, in some demonstrable respect, the welfare of those for whom the care is being provided, and although there will be some scope for 'customer choice', the role of the expertise of the providers is fundamental. (Note that this account is agnostic on whether state or market provision is best, for on this view it is largely a technical rather than a principled issue, i.e. it is a matter of discovering which does the job most efficiently and effectively.) At the risk of over-stating the case, on this view, 'care' is seen as a specialist service supplied by those who are trained to provide it to those who need it. The model here is clearly similar to that of modern scientific medicine understood as a relation between doctor (an expert and 'authority') and patient, the trusting and largely passive recipient of 'treatment'.

Now the validity of this model can be questioned even in relation to medicine; however, whatever its plausibility there, its appropriateness as a model for the provision of many other kinds of social care is still more contestable. (This is not to suggest, what is not the case, that there is a sharp distinction between health care and social care – clearly there is a very extensive grey area though this is not to deny either that there is a distinction (Griffiths, 1988; Department of Health, 1989). The most important reason for resisting what might be called the 'medical model' is that it pays insufficient attention to the character and quality of the relationship involved in caring, and it places too much emphasis on 'outcomes', narrowly conceived. This has its roots in a failure to take adequate account of the ineliminable subjective component of welfare. People's well-being is in part, only in part but none the less a significant part, a function of their own perception of, including their feelings about, their situation. An important feature of most people's judgements about the quality of their lives, is the nature of their relationships with other people. It matters a good deal to people how and why other people relate to them. This is not just a question of 'service with a smile', though no doubt that matters too, but also, and more significantly, about the value people attach to each other and their reasons for doing what they do.

It is helpful at this point to distinguish the argument being developed here from one increasingly voiced by some of the 'subjects' of care, especially the physically disabled (Oliver, 1990; Morris, 1993). They too are often critical of the role of professionals in defining their needs and determining how they are best met. A particular motivation underlying this response is the lack of control and choice that disabled people experience in relation to the professionals who are supposed to be assisting them. The ensuing argument, however, is rather different to this one, potentially though not necessarily in tension with it. It stresses the ineliminable role of mutual dependency in all our lives – the nature and extent obviously varying between individuals and situations – and contends that this should not be seen in exclusively negative terms. Of course, excessive dependency and lack of control over a long time can be distressing, and to this extent is something to be remedied wherever possible. But dependency, emotional and physical, is part of the human condition, and is not necessarily a cause for regret or something always to be avoided: it is one of the elements in life that binds human beings together. So, without wishing to deny the arguments for greater control and independence we should not expect too much in this direction, and it is far from obvious, for example, that seeking to make most relationships between carers and cared for essentially contractual, in the name of choice and control for the latter, would be an unmixed blessing.

Furthermore, in suggesting that some forms of social care are not best provided by professionals, it is important to understand that this is not a criticism of professionals. It is not that they are in some way failing to do what they should, but that there are some things they cannot do while maintaining a professional relationship with those for whom they provide care. For instance, professionals have an extensive range of obligations and responsibilities to the organizations that employ them; obligations and responsibilities determined by those organizations and the legal structure in which they operate. These obligations and responsibilities define and characterize the relationship between professional carers and those for whom they care. These relationships can be defined with more or less sensitivity and flexibility, but some such structure of obligations and responsibilities is both unavoidable and wholly appropriate. It is part of the accountability of such professionals, whether publicly or privately funded. Of course, actual relationships may, and do on occasion, exceed or differ from the parameters prescribed by the formal definition. However, in so far as they do so, the relationship to that extent ceases to be a professional one, and a qualitatively different relationship is established. This need not be objectionable, indeed if the 'extra' is provided at the cost (more likely time than money) of the professional then it may be admirable. However, when this happens it is indicative of a non-professional relationship, one for which the carer is not accountable to his or her employers (though if things go wrong the very fact that the person is a 'professional' may give rise to questions that would not be asked where the person had no professional obligations or code to observe).

Care by the Community

The conception of community care that I wish to articulate and defend has two distinctive components. First, it tries to 'demystify' social care by emphasizing the role of non-specialists and non-professionals. It draws attention to the kind of help that pretty much anyone is capable of providing, if willing to devote the necessary time and attention. Second, it locates the provision of care in certain sorts of practices, and social relationships within civil society. That is, it sees the provision of care as not exclusively the responsibility of the affected individual or of the state. It does not preclude, indeed it is entirely consistent with encouraging people to insure themselves against certain sorts of risks, and nor is it incompatible with a large role for the state, partly in fostering suitable arrangements (including off-setting some, if not all, of the costs borne by carers). Each of these components is explained in a little more detail below.

Much of the care that is currently provided through professionals and specialist organizations could be provided, at least in principle, by ordinary people, with at most a minimal level of 'training'. In the past, these often were, and to an underestimated extent still are, provided by family, kin, neighbours and friendly associations (Walker, 1986). (The diminished role within trades unions for the welfare functions, which often formed part of their original ethos, has been unfortunate both for the provision of welfare and for trades unions.) The care of older people; of young children; of those people with various milder forms of physical or mental disability; support for colleagues, friends or kin experiencing hardship, or personal crisis through the vicissitudes of unemployment or marital breakdown; the consequences of illness or injury and other forms of dislocation; and many other kinds of care frequently do not require much in the way of professional expertise. Indeed, the 'professionalization' of 'care' can too easily become an excuse for the reluctance of the rest of us to provide these types of support: we cannot do it because we are not 'qualified', and in any case it is not our responsibility. Instead people with such problems must be left to social workers, various sorts of therapists, marriage guidance counsellors or placed in homes or hospitals. Again, it must be emphasized that this is not to deny that there is a place for experts or for specialized institutions, but too often these can become a substitute for the care that ought to be a normal part of a variety of personal and informal social relations.

This leads naturally to the second component of this conception of community care, the role of civil society rather than exclusive concern with the alternatives of individual self-reliance or state provision. This dichotomy, which pervades much of the more ideologically motivated discussion of social care and welfare provision, is pernicious. In either of the extreme forms, it is simply misleading about the circumstances of human life. The emphasis upon individual self-reliance denies the extent to which we are all dependent on one another, and exaggerates the degree to which it is reasonable or desirable to expect people to protect themselves against all the harsher contingencies of life. There is nothing necessarily shameful or demeaning about needing the support and help of others, nor is it always unreasonable to be expected to provide such help and support when one is in a position to do so.

By contrast, the emphasis on the role of the state as a kind of surrogate parent – providing protection and support for every individual from cradle to grave – is both unrealistic in the demands it imposes on the state and potentially dangerously infantilizing. Part of attaining a level of personal maturity is taking on some significant degree of responsibility for our lives and not expecting to be rescued from the consequences of every misjudgment we make or every misfortune that befalls us. Again, this is not to deny an important place to both individual self-reliance and state provision, but it is to claim that there are, in addition, other important possibilities, possibilities that are all too easily neglected or overlooked in the debate between proponents of individual self-reliance and advocates of the all-encompassing welfare state.

These intermediate possibilities which comprise the case for community care, as outlined, draw on relationships that are less impersonal than those constituted by citizenship – at least if that is understood as an exclusively political identity. 'Community', despite its slipperiness and modishness at the present time, seems to be an appropriate term for capturing the kinds of values and qualities that it invokes. There is at best, only an attenuated sense in which a modern state can give effective expression to the values of community; for the state is largely a bureaucratic and legalistic framework of administration and control. Of course it should not, because of this, be undervalued: it is bound up with such fundamental values of the rule of law, equal citizenship and impartial justice. However, there are limits to what we can expect from it, and a modern state is not well designed to provide a locus for the kind of social care that typically grows out of smaller and more intimate groups. Similarly, the market is generally an unsuitable mechanism for providing such care. It too is impersonal in its operations, mediating relations through the cash nexus rather than any moral or emotional bonds. The market may be an entirely adequate structure for the provision of a wide range of consumer goods but it is not the sort of relationship on which the kinds of care that are of concern here can be satisfactorily built.

The values that community care invokes, therefore, are not ones that are easily expressed through the state or the market. They involve a sense of fellow-feeling and interconnectedness, which is simply not feasible at the level of the modern state, and in which the market does not deal. Community care requires specific relationships with particular others, which are largely constituted by affective bonds implying ethical commitments. These bonds need not be intense emotional relationships, but they do involve a level of concern for the other, that, when necessary, is sufficient to elicit a practical response. The provision of social care when it is needed is one way in which this will be expressed. In these relationships there is no formal division between carer and cared for; no structure of authority; and no clear specification of exactly what is to be provided, on what terms and at what cost. These can only be emergent features of particular situations, in which much will depend upon the precise circumstances. Undoubtedly this will make for an element of unpredictability in the distribution of care, but this is likely under even the most formalized and comprehensive system of provision. In any case, it is not suggested that community care will not need to be supplemented by other forms of provision.

Objections to Community Care

To conclude, and in the process elaborate a little further on this defence of one ideal of community care, two important objections will be examined, though these do not exhaust the potential problems. Both of these objections raise serious problems, especially the second, but they do not seem to be obviously insuperable. Nor do they invalidate the ideal of community care, though they do suggest a certain caution about any too exclusive and uncritical pursuit of it.

The first objection is that the burden of community care, as it has been described, will in fact fall disproportionately on already disadvantaged members of society. Women are likely to shoulder a disproportionate share, so too, probably, will the poor, and as Atkin suggests in this volume, members of ethnic minority groups. Thus, it will be argued that community care is likely to be inequitable, and exacerbate existing inequalities, rather than redistribute resources from the wealthy to the needy. There is little doubt that this is what would happen (and is in fact happening) if state provision was simply withdrawn. However, this is not what has been suggested. Community care is quite consistent with, indeed ideally needs to be fostered by, policies that make its provision through the kinds of social relationships described here more feasible and less burdensome. This can be encouraged through a range of financial provisions, including manipulation of the tax system, and by other measures that facilitate the flourishing of smaller groups, and promote the formation of reciprocal relationships of concern and support. These financial provisions are unlikely to remove all the sting from this objection, but they could significantly weaken it.

However, this first objection also clearly reveals how attitudes have to change. It refers exclusively to the *burdens* of providing care, and of course it is important not to sentimentalize what is involved. Often, that will be unavoidably burdensome, requiring time-consuming and sometimes unpleasant tasks. But, is this *all* there is to provision of such care? Does it not tell us something significant, and not very admirable about our attitudes to others – that caring should be thought of exclusively as a burden? Are there no rewards, is there no sense of satisfaction to be gained from helping our neighbours, kin, friends, colleagues or whoever? If the answer really is an unequivocal no then it does seem that there is little hope for the sort of community care previously sketched out. It is unlikely that people who feel this way would ever be sufficiently motivated to undertake community care (though it is equally unlikely that they can be persuaded to support a generous level of welfare provision by the state). However, is it right to be so pessimistic?

This last point hints at the second objection to be considered. That is, to slightly adapt a famous remark of Mrs Thatcher's, that there is no such thing as community. It might be argued, even by those sympathetic to the ideal of community care, that the institutions and relationships which comprise the 'community' are too attenuated to perform the robust role here assigned them. Moreover, there is no reason to think that they can be wished into existence merely because they are thought to be desirable. A good example of this is kinship, the kind of locally-based, extended kinship networks that were commonplace in the past, and which, among poorer sections of society, often provided invaluable forms of social support, such as child-care and help for aged or infirm relatives, but are now a rarity. Smaller families, greater labour mobility, and a variety of other social effects of late capitalism, have all combined to winnow away at extended kinship networks, and have done so for reasons that suggest that this trend is pretty much irreversible. We cannot look, therefore, to what does not exist and cannot be made to exist, for the provision of social care. Many people will simply not belong to groups or have relationships with other people able and willing to provide the support they need and on which the practical effectiveness of this conception of community care depends.

This is an objection that must be taken very seriously; it is an objection that, if it goes through, ultimately undermines the entire feasibility, whatever its desirability in the abstract, of the ideal of community care. Again, the question that must be asked is whether the situation is, or need be, quite so hopeless as this objection maintains. Certainly, the objection is a strong one in relation to extended kinship networks but is it so powerful in relation to neighbours, friends, voluntary associations and other informal groups? Is it inconceivable to think, for example, that neighbourhood watch schemes, at present concerned exclusively with the protection of property, could be transformed into neighbourhood support schemes, addressing a wider range of needs? It is not obvious that the situation is without possibilities, and interestingly enough, both the moderate left and the moderate right have been concerned of late to stress the importance of strengthening and developing the institutions and relations of civil society in arguments for the social market or civic capitalism (Green, 1993).

Conclusion

As hopefully is clear, the suggestion of this chapter is not that community care should be seen as a panacea to all our problems of social care. Nor is it that self-reliance and state provision do not have a large and ineliminable role to play in the provision of welfare, including social care. Without significant levels of self-reliance the expectations generated of social care would be excessively demanding. The state, too, will always be necessary where self-reliance and community care fail, as they always will, in some circumstances and for some people. What I have tried to argue is that community care can also play an important part in promoting welfare if it is understood, not simply as a cost-cutting exercise, but as a more deeply rooted aspiration towards mutuality expressed through a variety of relationships and small-scale organizations which connect people one to another.

It is to be hoped that the disrepute in which the current policy of community care is widely held does not carry over to all ideals of reposing more responsibility for social care outside the simple duality of individual self-reliance and state provision. The issues are too important for the ideal of community care to be ceded wholesale to Treasury cost-cutters with an eye to a quick fix.

References

BULMER, M. (1987) *Social Basis of Community Care*, London: Allen and Unwin.
CHALLIS D. and HUGMAN R. (1993) 'Editorial: community care, social work, and social care', *British Journal of Social Work*, **23**(4), pp. 319–28.
DEPARTMENT OF HEALTH (1989) *Caring for People: Community Care in the Next Decade and Beyond*, Cm 849, London: HMSO.
GREEN D. (1993) *Reinventing Civil Society: The Rediscovery of Welfare Without Politics*,

London: IEA Health and Welfare Unit.

GRIFFITHS, R. (1988) *Community Care: Agenda for Action*, Londc

MORRIS, J. (1993) *Independent Lives? Community Care and Dis*
   stoke: Macmillan.

OLIVER, M. (1990) *The Politics of Disablement*, London: Macmillaı

PARKER, G. (1990) *With Due Care and Attention: A Review of R*   ..ul
   Care, 2nd Edn., London: Family Policy Studies Centre.

TWIGG, J. and ATKIN, K. (1994) *Carers Perceived: Policy and Practice in Informal Care*,
   Buckingham: Open University Press.

WALKER A. (1986) 'Community care: fact and fiction', in WILMOTT, P. (Ed.) *The Debate
   About Community: Papers from a Seminar on 'Community Care and Social Policy'*,
   London: Policy Studies Institute.

New Issues

Chapter 8

Contracting Welfare? Market Testing and Social Security[1]

Roy Sainsbury and Steven Kennedy

Introduction

... competition is good for the *users* of public services. It gives them a
wider variety of facilities and services. Competition is good for *taxpayers*,
who get better value for their money. It is good for *managers*, who can
concentrate on their core activities. It is good for *staff*, who can give their
best in a more competitive environment. And it is good for *business*,
giving private firms new opportunities to market their services.

> (HM Treasury, 1991: foreword by Norman Lamont,
> emphasis in original)

Major structural changes have been introduced by the separation of institutions
into buyers and sellers, and the introduction of competitive tendering. It is now
time to evaluate the implementation of these structural changes through the
process of working out new ways of relating within the structures. The simplistic
economic transaction being the single solution to all relationships will not do
(Flynn, 1993, p. 3).

In November 1991, the Government published its White Paper *Competing
for Quality* (HM Treasury, 1991), in which it outlined plans for 'market testing'
in the public sector. The market testing proposals, which were presented as part
of the 'Citizen's Charter' initiative, are, according to the Government, aimed at
achieving greater value for money whilst improving the quality of service
provided by Government departments and agencies.

This chapter examines market testing as it affects the administration of
social security. As indicated by the opening quotation, competitive tendering in
the public sector is advocated for a variety of reasons, but the main focus of this
chapter is on the consequences of market testing for social security claimants
themselves. It begins by describing the market testing programme of the

Department of Social Security (DSS), and the more *ad hoc* developments in the local authority sector. The discussion that follows considers the arguments put forward for market testing, and explores some of the problems raised by the introduction of competitive tendering in social security administration. Finally, it is considered how the DSS market testing programme might evolve.

What is Market Testing?

Before describing the extent of the market testing programme in social security, we should be clear about what market testing is, and how it relates to privatization. In a speech to representatives of the private sector in the spring of 1993, William Waldegrave, the then Citizen's Charter Minister, clearly set out the Government's thinking behind its approach to exposing the public sector to the rigours of the market. In brief, he explained that public services should be carefully scrutinized to determine whether they should be provided at all. If a public service survives this test, then ideally it should be sold to the private sector. This is privatization in its pure, undiluted form. If, however, it is decided that overall responsibility for providing the service should remain in the public sector, then the service should be contracted out directly to the private sector. However, if there are doubts about whether the private sector can undertake the function more cost-effectively, then in-house teams should also be invited to submit tenders to run the service. It is this last option which is referred to as 'market testing'. It is clear from the Waldegrave speech that these choices form a definite hierarchy. The message to Government departments can therefore be reduced to a simple catechism:

1   If it is *not* required, then abolish it.
2   If it *is* required, can it be sold off?
3   If it cannot be sold off, can it be contracted out directly?
4   If none of these is possible, then consider market testing.

What the Waldegrave catechism appears to imply is that the market testing programme is part of a wider strategy, which sees the minimization of the role of the state as the primary objective. We return to this issue later, since we believe it is of crucial importance in understanding both the Government's motives behind these reforms and the possible direction of future developments.

The DSS Market Testing Programme

Before the market testing programme came into operation, the DSS was already spending about half of its £2 billion annual running costs, and nearly all of its £350 million capital funds, with private sector contractors. Of this, over £500 million was being spent on the procurement of services (HM Treasury, 1991).

In 1991/2, the DSS began nine 'tests' involving around £50 million worth of services. The first year of the programme proper began in 1992, with the announcement of market testing plans for 28 service areas encompassing DSS headquarters and all five of its executive agencies. The Benefits Agency (BA) alone was to test 15 operations. The total value of this business was, at that time, put at £127 million, and the programme was to be completed by September 1993.

The programme included some of the usual candidates for contracting out (such as accommodation and office services, catering, printing, and storage and distribution) and some other, relatively obscure activities (such as video production, microfilming, and travel services), though none of these was concerned directly with the delivery of benefits to claimants. However, there were also activities earmarked for testing that impinged much more directly on the claiming population. Included in the programme were debt recovery and the Benefits Agency Medical Service (whose staff of medical officers carry out assessments and provide reports for those benefits requiring medical input, such as sickness benefit and invalidity benefit[2]). Fraud investigation, although not included in the published plans, was also considered.

The programme did not, however, keep to its original timetable. Of the 28 areas announced in the 1992/3 programme only six (three of which were linked to the Benefits Agency but were small specialist services only) had gone through the full market testing or contracting out process. At the end of the year 1992/3, the total value of the business market tested amounted to only £15 million (compared with the £127 million target). The DSS was not alone in falling behind. Fewer than 200 of the 350 departmental functions across Whitehall due to be market tested by September 1993 were completed. However, figures released by the Cabinet Office show that the DSS had by far the worst record of all departments in terms of the proportion of the total target value of business actually disposed of (*Guardian*, 6 August 1994).

Officials involved in the market testing programme point towards the sheer size and complexity of the task as part of the reason for falling so far behind target. In addition, they were hampered by delays in receiving central guidance about how to conduct market testing from the Government's Efficiency Unit. Another cause of the delay in the market testing programme, not only in the DSS but throughout Whitehall, was the legal uncertainty surrounding the applicability of the European Union's 'Acquired Rights Directive 1981', (which was implemented in Britain as the Transfer of Undertakings (Protection of Employment) Regulations 1981). The directive aims to protect the terms and conditions of workers whose jobs are transferred to new employers, but there has been considerable disagreement as to whether it applies to civil servants whose positions are threatened by market testing and contracting out. A further reason for delay, which also has wider significance, was that, in the process of market testing, other means of disposing of services arose in some areas. Most notably, having begun the market testing process, staff at BA Publishing proposed a management buy-out as an alternative. This bid was successful, and therefore sets a challenging precedent for the rest of the Benefits Agency.

So far, we have discussed market testing only in relation to the DSS. However, two of the main means-tested benefits, housing benefit and council tax benefit, are administered not by the Benefits Agency but by local authorities. Local authorities have long been able to adapt how they deliver these benefits to their own administrative structures and, to a degree, to political imperatives. Furthermore, local Government has been used to competitive tendering and contracting out for many years, though benefit administration has remained largely untouched by privatization until recently.

It is only in the last two years that the private sector has gained a foothold in benefit administration. By January 1994, four local authorities had directly contracted out the administration of housing and council tax benefit to the same private company (no in-house bids were sought). Housing benefits staff are now employees of the private company, not the local authority. Their role is to prepare claims for decision by a council officer. They do not make decisions themselves; decisions on benefit eligibility remain the responsibility of the council. Any potential difficulties arising from private sector workers making decisions that effectively distribute central Government monies are therefore avoided, at least in theory. Service level agreements have been drawn up, specifying, for example, target clearance times and standards of service for claimants. The company is responsible for all equipment and running costs. Staff have been able to retain their local authority terms and conditions of service or opt for a new contract with the company.

Little attention has been paid to these developments in housing and council tax benefit administration, despite their radical nature. As far as the authors are aware, no independent research has as yet been carried out into the impact of these changes. At present we do not know what effect contracting out has had on the decisions made on housing benefit claims. For example, has benefit expenditure increased or decreased? Has the number of overpayments or backdated awards changed? What sort of decisions are being made about restricted rents? What is happening to exceptional circumstances payments? Has the time spent on advising claimants or explaining decisions been reduced? Are there other aspects of service that have been cut back in favour of pushing claims through the system? Despite these unanswered questions, the expansion of the private sector in local authority benefit administration appears to be quickening.

These developments have not, however, gone unnoticed by central Government. In an article in the DSS internal newsletter, *Market Testing* (issue 16), it is revealed that the 'Benefits Administration Review' currently under way in the DSS will investigate the experience of local authorities that have contracted out the housing benefit delivery process. If the outcome of this review is favourable, the next few years could see the extension of the DSS programme beyond the mainly peripheral activities market tested so far, to the more sensitive areas of benefits administration that constitute the 'core business' of the DSS and its agencies. The remainder of this chapter considers the consequences for social security claimants of such a scenario, beginning by examining in greater depth the case put forward for market testing.

The Case for Market Testing

The proponents of market testing argue that the introduction of competition and contracts in the provision of public services would result in both greater value for money and better quality services. Efficiency improvements, it is claimed, result from three main sources. First, the process of inviting bids from prospective operators provides managers with alternative cost estimates for providing a particular service (Chaundy and Uttley, 1993). Such information may not have been available previously. Second, the possibility of not being awarded the contract to provide a particular service (or losing the contract, in the case of existing suppliers), encourages organizations to submit tenders at minimum cost. Where services were previously delivered by a single monopoly supplier, it is claimed, such incentives did not exist. Third, the introduction of built-in competitive pressures reduces the possibility of bureaucratic expansion, which, according to public choice theorists, is an inherent problem with monopoly public sector organizations (see for example, Niskanen, 1971).

Improvements in service quality, according to the proponents of market testing, also occur as a result of competitive tendering. This occurs partly as a result of the separation of policy specification from service delivery. According to Mather (1991), traditional hierarchical public sector bureaucracies are characterized by a 'conflict of interest' that is to the detriment of service users. This view also permeates the *Competing for Quality* White Paper. The 'old approach', according to the Government, created 'a culture that was more often concerned with procedures than performance' (HM Treasury, 1991). Splitting the process of service level specification from service provision, and introducing competition, it is argued, removes this conflict of interest and allows a refocussing of attention away from the interests of service providers towards the needs of users. Moreover, the introduction of monitoring procedures to ensure suppliers comply with the terms of the contract create a built-in pressure to maintain the improved standards of service. Thus, according to the proponents of market testing, there is an increased emphasis on the quality of service provided.

These arguments are compelling, and indeed initial evidence from developments so far in social security administration do appear to suggest that the reforms are resulting in at least some of the expected benefits. With regard to efficiency improvements, it is as yet too early to gauge the magnitude of any financial effects, but preliminary evidence from the contracting out of housing benefit administration suggests that there is potential for cost savings.

Although cost savings are an important consideration with market testing, the impact of the initiative on the quality and nature of the 'services' provided is perhaps of greater relevance for social security recipients. Anecdotal evidence of how the reforms are proceeding, in this respect, does appear encouraging. According to officials involved in the market testing initiative, the splitting up of the DSS bureaucracy has forced managers of service areas to examine what they do, why and how they do it, and at what cost, often for the first time. Those who are 'purchasing' services have also been required to specify what standard of service they want, and at what price. In this way, therefore, market testing may be forcing another change, after 'Next Steps', in the culture within the DSS.

It should be remembered, however, that within the DSS, the market testing programme, so far, has largely been limited to activities where the 'customer' is another branch of the DSS itself; where the 'product' in question is relatively easy to define, and where 'quality' is relatively easy to measure. In most cases the service areas market tested are similar to activities that are commonly contracted out in private sector organizations. Storage and printing services, for example, both of which were included in the Benefits Agency 1992/3 market testing programme, are similar to commercial enterprises. If market testing is extended beyond such relatively straightforward activities and into areas that involve the processing of claims and the delivery of benefits, however, the issues that need to be addressed become somewhat more complex, and the advantages for claimants less certain.

To elaborate, it is necessary first to consider the nature of the 'service' being provided, the 'customer' whose interests are being considered, the aims and objectives for the service, and the ability to identify what is meant by 'quality', in the context of benefits administration. Consider, for example, the processing of claims for, and the payment of, income support. From the perspective of *social security claimants*, the most important factor is undoubtedly the level of benefit itself and the conditions of entitlement. However, it is clear that choices with respect to factors such as these will remain political choices. The areas of concern are therefore somewhat more limited, relating to the process of dealing with benefit claims and the way in which benefit is paid. For claimants, factors such as the quick processing of claims, the provision of advice and information relating to eligibility, courteous and non-intrusive treatment by staff, and regular payment of benefit may be important considerations. Claimants however are not the only group with an interest in benefit administration. For the Government itself, the minimization of administration costs is obviously an important objective, reflecting public expenditure concerns. In addition, Ministers might also be concerned with ensuring effective procedures to detect fraud, not only because of the expenditure implications but also because of political priorities.

Welfare rights organizations and other pressure groups can also be expected to express an interest in aspects of social security administration. For such groups, the take-up of benefits, open and fair procedures, and the maintenance of effective means of redress for dissatisfied claimants, are likely to be key areas of interest. Many of these concerns may also be shared by the general public themselves, who might also be concerned that the system reflects wider notions of social justice. As taxpayers, the public might also share the Government's interest in ensuring that resources are more effectively 'targeted' on those most in need.

From the discussion above, it is clear that the aims and objectives of social security administration can be both numerous and, potentially, conflicting. As a consequence, the outcome of market testing sensitive areas of the benefit system could potentially be detrimental for claimants. In part, this is due to the problems associated with applying the 'contract model' in such circumstances.

Government by Contract?

The case for market testing and contracting out rests crucially on the implicit assumption that contracts *are* an appropriate mechanism to regulate relationships in the public sector. The literature on the problems and pitfalls of contracting is large (see for example, Vickers and Yarrow, 1988; Flynn, 1994). However, what is clear from the literature is that there are a number of prerequisites that must be met if contracts are to be applied in an unproblematic manner. First, purchasers of services must be able to specify service requirements clearly. Second, the contract must fully encapsulate all aspects of service needs. Third, the purchaser must be able to monitor accurately the performance of the contractor to ensure that the terms of the contract are not being broken and that targets are being met. Finally, the purchaser must have recourse to effective means of redress if the terms of the contract are not satisfied.

From the previous discussion, it is clear that many areas of social security administration fall short of these requirements in a number of respects. In the case of processing claims for income support, for example, it is doubtful that a workable contract could be drawn up that incorporated every aspect of 'performance' of concern to all the relevant stakeholders. Even if it were possible to state clearly the service requirements, it is by no means certain that the authorities could effectively monitor all aspects of the behaviour of the contractor to ensure that the terms of the contract were being adhered to. The DSS and its agencies have made considerable progress in recent years in developing more relevant and reliable performance indicator systems (Carter and Greer, 1993). However, what is becoming increasingly clear from the literature is that there are limits to what can be measured accurately in the public sector, and that consequently performance indicators, although useful, should be regarded merely as one element of a wider process of performance assessment, one which also incorporates more subtle judgements and opinions (Stewart and Walsh, 1994).

The extent to which problems with contracts occur of course depends upon the nature of the service in question. More routine operations, where procedures are dictated by clear and explicit sets of rules (such as, for example, the collection of National Insurance contributions), may be more amenable to the contract model. However, in many areas of social security administration the activity in question is considerably more complex, and may involve officials exercising discretionary powers (for example, decisions by Child Support Agency officials about which cases to pursue). Issues such as these may indeed prove problematic given the apparent trend towards a 'discretionary' welfare state (the substitution of the Social Fund for the previous system of single payments is perhaps the most obvious manifestation of this trend, but also relevant are the proposals to tighten up the 'actively seeking work' rules with the introduction of the 'Jobseeker's Allowance').

The crucial point to be made, which some advocates of the 'contracting state' (for example, Mather, 1991) fail to recognize, is that 'performance' in many areas of the public sector is by no means a simple concept to grasp. Given this, the possibility exists that the extension of market testing to certain areas of the DSS could be detrimental for social security claimants. It is not unrealistic to imagine a scenario where a contractor, faced with the task of meeting a limited number of inadequate (probably financial) performance targets, allows other 'softer' aspects of service, which may be of more importance to claimants, to deteriorate.

Values and Stakeholders

Even if the problems surrounding the introduction of the competitive tendering of sensitive services were resolved, it is still by no means certain that claimants would benefit. For while market testing purports to solve the 'problem' of market failure in the provision of public services, its proponents are strangely silent on another important issue that is of direct relevance: the possible failure of Government itself to reflect the aspirations and preferences of those for whom services are provided. The market testing initiative is, like an earlier DSS organizational initiative, the *Operational Strategy*, a 'top-down' reform (see Adler and Sainsbury, 1991), and similarly runs the risk of reflecting the priorities of Government itself to the exclusion of other legitimate stakeholders.

Clearly, much depends on whether the concerns of claimants and groups campaigning on their behalf are given adequate prominence in the market testing initiative. Thus far however, little, if any, attempt has been made to elicit the views of either of these important 'stakeholders' in the market testing process, at least explicitly. Indeed, in the introduction to the first issue of the DSS internal newsletter, *Market Testing*, Peter Lilley does not even mention social security claimants, but stresses his overriding concern to deliver 'value for money for taxpayers'.

The DSS market testing programme to date has, however, mainly concentrated on areas that are of little direct interest for the claiming population, so it is possible to argue that the concerns outlined above are not relevant, at least at present. Nevertheless, given the likelihood that the market testing initiative will be extended to more sensitive areas of the benefits system, the importance of these considerations remains.

How might the interests of the various stakeholders be incorporated into the market testing process? One possibility would be to ask social security claimants themselves. The creation of executive agencies such as the Benefits Agency has, undeniably, been accompanied by increasing emphasis on the 'quality' of service provided; and much effort has gone into 'customer' surveys and the like to elicit the views of claimants on many aspects of the benefit delivery system. However, at present there is no requirement for Government to act on the findings of such surveys. Clearly, what is needed is some mechanism to ensure that the interests of claimants and their representatives are given prominence. A possible model for this is suggested by recent changes in New Zealand, where the reorganization of Government departments along agency lines (not unlike the changes introduced in the UK in the late 1980s) was accompanied by the establishment of public bodies to represent the interests of certain disadvantaged groups. These bodies, which include Women's Affairs and Youth Affairs agencies, were set up specifically to ensure that groups with limited institutional influence could have a more effective input into the policymaking process, particularly in areas of Government activity where there are potentially conflicting objectives (Boston, 1991).

Yet another more radical option relates to the 'Citizen's Charter' initiative, with its emphasis on 'empowerment' for the users of public services. Before outlining some of the policy options, it is first necessary, however, to look at the theoretical arguments underpinning the Citizen's Charter.

Empowerment and Choice

The market testing initiative itself was originally presented as part of the Citizen's Charter initiative, and many of the advocates of competitive tendering have emphasized the potential for new arrangements to offer individuals greater powers in relation to public services. For example, Mather (1991) argues that

it [the contract model] is compatible with specific remedies and new enforcement powers for individuals who have suffered loss by reason of

Government failure, or the failure of agencies granted monopoly or other enhanced powers by the state.

Mather's argument is that the 'transparency' of contracts results in the 'empowerment' of individual citizens since they have a clear idea of what standard of service to expect, and the specific means to seek redress if these standards are not met.

As far as the market testing programme in the DSS is concerned, there has been little mention so far of the possibility of granting individual 'customers' means of redress if the service they receive is inadequate. This may in part reflect the emphasis on cost saving, which has been the primary motivation behind the reforms. It also reflects the fact that the relationship between the individual claimant and the agencies responsible for assessing eligibility for and delivering benefits is different in a number of respects to the relationship between producers and consumers in other areas of the public and private sectors. In social security, the relationship can involve elements of coercion, stigma, and (increasingly) the use of discretion on the part of officials. Given these realities, in many areas of social security administration the notion of 'rights' to a particular standard of service is less meaningful than in most other public services. Nevertheless, many of the activities carried out in the administration of social security are amenable to the application of the Citizen's Charter principle. Although administrative machinery required to put this into operation would inevitably be cumbersome, it is notable that many organizations in the private sector that perform similar functions (for example, banks) have themselves introduced customer charters.

A more radical alternative would be to recognize the importance of *choice* for social security claimants. On first reflection, it might appear that there is little potential for individual claimants to exercise choice within the current system. However, many core DSS activities are at present conducted in local benefit offices, and if the DSS were to contract out benefits administration on an office-by-office basis (rather than contracting out each function nationally or regionally), then it might be possible to offer claimants the possibility of choosing which office would deal with their claim. The degree of choice might be constrained by geographical considerations, but given the potential of computerization, even this constraint may disappear. There is some opportunity, therefore, at least theoretically, for market testing to lead to the empowerment of social security claimants.

Conclusion

The market testing initiative has been presented as having something for everyone. Users of services benefit, managers benefit, staff benefit, and the private sector benefits. However, we would argue that the case for market testing many activities in the social security system is by no means as clear as the Government suggests.

Closer examination of how the DSS market testing programme has progressed so far suggests that the Government may be waking up to some of its problems, and that consequently the scope for market testing may be somewhat more limited than was initially envisaged. It now appears that functions that involve decisions with regard to individual claims, adjudication, and compelling individuals to attend benefit offices, are not to be market tested, though DSS officials stress that there are no legal obstacles to contracting out the administrative 'spade work' surrounding these activities (*Market Testing*, Issue 7). In this context, it is interesting to note that after some two years of feasibility studies and reviews, Benefits Agency officials announced that the market testing of fraud investigation was 'inappropriate at this time' (*Market Testing*, Issue 19). Similar delays have occurred in announcing the plans for the Benefits Agency Medical Services, and it remains to be seen whether the Agency will press on with the market testing of debt recovery services. More recent pronouncements suggest that throughout Whitehall there may be less emphasis on market testing and contracting out than was the case previously, with individual departments being given greater freedom to adopt alternative measures such as efficiency scrutinies or internal reviews. In addition, 'prior options' reviews will now occur once every five years rather than every three years as originally envisaged (*Market Testing*, Issue 20).[3] It would appear, therefore, that the goal of 'government by contract' may prove somewhat more elusive than its proponents suggest.

The case for introducing competitive tendering in social security administration, as in other areas of the public sector, is predicated on a particular view of public administration, which assumes that it is possible to restructure the public sector in such a way as to separate the political function of service specification and the technical or administrative processes involved in delivering those services. However, we would argue that this approach is simplistic, and ignores many of the realities that distinguish many activities in the public sphere from the private sector. We believe that, unless many of the issues discussed are considered, the market testing programme may do nothing for social security claimants and, indeed, could result in a deterioration in the 'quality of service' experienced by some of the most vulnerable groups in society.

It would be churlish, however, to dismiss entirely the case for introducing competitive tendering in social security administration. If nothing else, the market testing initiative raises very important questions about what the goals of social security should be, how it should be organized, whose interests should be taken into account, and how to measure 'performance'. Market testing could turn out to be a useful exercise in helping to determine the future shape of the social security system, to the benefit of all the relevant stakeholders – claimants as well as taxpayers and the Government. Unfortunately, the primary motivation behind the initiative so far has been the curtailment of public expenditure and the minimization of the role of the state.

Market testing will only succeed in its stated aims if it is recognized that 'quality' in the provision of public sector services is as much an important consideration as economy.

Notes

1   This chapter is an expanded and revised version of an article that appeared originally in *Benefits* (Sainsbury and Kennedy, 1994).
2   Invalidity benefit was replaced by a new benefit, incapacity benefit, in April 1995.
3   'Prior options' reviews set the priorities for the agency in the short term.

References

ADLER, M. and SAINSBURY, R. (1991) 'The social shaping of information technology: computerisation and the administration of social security', in ADLER, M., BELL, C., CLASEN, J. and SINFIELD, A. (Eds) *The Sociology of Social Security*, Edinburgh: Edinburgh University Press.

BOSTON, J. (1991) 'Reorganizing the machinery of government: Objectives and outcomes', in BOSTON, J., MARTIN, J., PALLOT, J. and WALSH, P. (Eds) *Reshaping the State: New Zealand's Bureaucratic Revolution*, Auckland: Oxford University Press.

CARTER, N. and GREER, P. (1993) 'Evaluating agencies: Next Steps and performance indicators', *Public Administration*, **71**, pp. 407–16.

CHAUNDY, D. and UTTLEY, M. (1993) 'The economics of compulsory competitive tendering: Issues, evidence and the case of municipal refuse collection', *Public Policy and Administration*, **8**(2), pp. 25–41.

FLYNN, N. (1993) 'Editorial: New management relationships in the public sector', *Public Money and Management*, September, p. 3.

FLYNN, N. (1994) 'Control, commitment and contracts', in CLARKE, J., COCHRANE, A. and MCLAUGHLIN, E. (Eds) *Managing Social Policy*, London: Sage.

HM TREASURY (1991) *Competing for Quality*, London: HMSO.

MATHER, G. (1991) 'Government by contract', in VIBERT, F. (Ed.) *Britain's Constitutional Future*, IEA Readings No. 36, London: Institute of Economic Affairs.

NISKANEN, W. (1971) *Bureaucracy and Representative Government*, Chicago: Aldine Atherton.

SAINSBURY, R. and KENNEDY, S. (1994) 'Flogging Social Security', *Benefits*, **10**, April/May, pp. 10–14.

STEWART, J. and WALSH, K. (1994) 'Performance measurement: When performance can never be finally defined', *Public Money and Management*, April–June, pp. 45–9.

VICKERS, J. and YARROW, G. (1988) *Privatisation: An Economic Analysis*, London: Massachusetts Institute of Technology Press.

Chapter 9

Accountability in Public Services: Incorporating the Professional Domain

Jane Lightfoot

Professional Accountability: A Neglected Domain

Accountability is a complex phenomenon. This is particularly so in modern democratic societies, given the range of agencies that exist to execute the affairs of state (Johnson, 1974; Day and Klein, 1987). It follows that any traditional notion of a simple accountability relationship between those in elected office and 'the people' is increasingly difficult to sustain. Indeed, much current interest in accountability stems from difficulties with control of public agencies; that is, how to ensure that 'political leaders and the public persuade, cajole or force administrative agencies to do their bidding' (Peters, 1989, p. 250).

At the heart of this analysis is an assumption that accountability can be divided into two broad domains: public–political and administrative–managerial (see for example, New, 1993). Political accountability takes place in a realm in which criteria for judging action are contestable. In other words, those with delegated authority from the people must give a 'persuasive account' for their actions (Day and Klein, 1987, p. 8). Administrative accountability, on the other hand, is a technical exercise in policy implementation. This classical model of accountability is characterized most clearly in the relationship between politicians and civil servants, with the work of the latter controlled within hierarchical, bureaucratic, organizations. This model might now be challenged on the grounds that it fails to reflect the changing nature of public agencies, in terms of the drive for increasing efficiency and flexibility through operation at arm's length from Government (Jenkins *et al.*, 1988).

In terms of this chapter, a more fundamental drawback of the classical model of accountability is that it obscures a third domain – that of the professional. Adopting special codes of behaviour and horizontal peer review (rather than the vertical lines of a bureaucracy), professional accountability does not sit comfortably within the classical model. While some writers acknowledge the existence of professionals within public organizations – and indeed record their threat to the classical model of control – professional accountability is portrayed as something of an anomaly, rather than as central to any debate about accountability relationships.

Peters (1989) cites the existence of professional employees as a 'common problem straining administrative control', since professionals have values that can conflict with those of the agency for which they work. Despite going so far as to suggest that this is an instance in which 'normal procedures of control and accountability may simply not be applicable', he recommends only 'some accommodation of values . . . perhaps on both sides' (Peters, 1989, p. 276).

Johnson suggests that professions adopt a confrontational stance to other systems for securing accountability:

> We ought to recognise . . . realistically that bureaucracies consist of clusters of interest . . . which may conspire against various modes of control and accountability intended to serve the interests of citizens. (Johnson, 1974, p. 8)

While acknowledging the impact on the classical model of accountability of the different perspective of professions, Johnson, like Peters, appears nevertheless ambivalent about analysing these conflicts directly. Yet relegating a consideration of professional accountability to the margins of analysis would seem not just an oversight, but also a serious weakening of the power of the classical model to explain accountability relationships in public services. This point is brought out particularly clearly by Day and Klein (1987) following their comparison of accountability across five public agencies:

> The debate and developments of the past two decades are, in retrospect, curiously lopsided. They revolve around the role of experts in accountability . . . But they neglect the accountability *of* experts. For one of the characteristics of service providers . . . is precisely that they tend to regard themselves as accountable to their peers and are thus not linked into the institutionalised system through which political and managerial accountability flow. (Day and Klein, 1987, p. 52, emphasis in original)

The assumption underlying this chapter is that any framework of accountability in public services requires that closer attention be given to incorporating the dimension of professional accountability. The purpose of such attention is to gain a fuller understanding of the relationship between professional, managerial and wider political, or public, elements of accountability, including identifying potential conflict between these elements and possibilities for reconciliation.

At the heart of this analysis is an examination of where power lies in controlling what Day and Klein (1987) term the 'language of evaluation'; that is, power to shape the meaning of accountability in practice (Day and Klein, 1987, p. 241). In other words, to what extent can and does professional autonomy dictate which values and activities are perceived as appropriate? Recent evidence indicates that, while professionals traditionally have enjoyed a good deal of autonomy (see for example, Lipsky, 1980; Wilding, 1982; Dalley, 1991; Hugman, 1991), the extent of such professional power is now challenged increasingly from both managers and consumers (Harrison, 1988a; Harrison *et al.*, 1989; Elston, 1991). In turn, these developments suggest that a contemporary analysis of professional accountability needs to be set in the context of attempts to assert control by non-professionals over professional work.

This chapter is neither a direct analysis of policy, nor an explicit contribution to the development of theory. Rather, it lies somewhere between the two as an attempt to draw attention to the importance of the professional domain as part of the framework of accountability in public services, with implications for both policy and theory.

The NHS professional and accountability

A consideration of the accountability of professionals in the National Health Service is particularly meaningful, since, in the UK, the doctrine of 'clinical freedom' has meant that health professionals (especially doctors) have traditionally enjoyed the capacity to shape patterns of health service provision. Historically, as Harrison (1988b) notes, health service administrators performed a 'diplomat' role, designed to support clinical practice within a framework of management by consensus.

In the early 1980s, the report of the enquiry into NHS management led by Roy Griffiths (Department of Health and Social Security, 1983) heralded a very different ideological approach, which was based upon executive power being held by a new breed of general managers appointed on the basis of managerial, rather than professional, skills. Implemented from 1985, this 'new managerialism' strengthened managerial accountability at the expense of professional accountability, through enhancing the manager role from that of supporting 'diplomat' to controlling 'agent' of central Government (Harrison, 1988b). Such a shift was reinforced by the rigours of the internal market introduced in 1991, for example through increased attention to cost reduction and improvements in efficiency, together with an emphasis on quality.

In an analysis of the extent of managerial control over health professionals, Harrison and Pollitt (1994) argue that the quest for this control has been seen by the Government as *the* solution to the management problems of the NHS. In turn, this belief rests upon a comparison of the extent of professional power compared with that of the private sector: 'After all, in ICI or Dupont or McDonnell-

Douglas there are plenty of professional experts but they are "on tap" for management, not "on top".' (Pollitt, 1993, p. 131)

A Framework of Accountability for NHS Professionals

So far, it has been argued that we can perceive NHS professionals as subject both to professional and managerial accountability. A further influence is the broader political context of public accountability for the NHS as a whole. Professional accountability in its simplest terms might be described by two key relationships: first, that between the professional and the individual patient or client; and, second, the relationship between the individual professional and a largely peer-governed professional body, responsible for standards and discipline.

The wider accountability framework within which NHS professionals operate incorporates both managerial and political accountability. In contrast to the emphasis within professional accountability on individual relationships, managerial accountability is characterized by a focus on matters of broad resource allocation, regularity, efficiency and effectiveness. Mechanisms for strengthening managerial accountability in the NHS have grown since the early 1980s, for example, performance indicators, efficiency savings and resource management (NHSME, 1991; Levitt and Wall, 1992). These changes have brought a sharper focus, on both the dual nature of accountability of professionals – to their profession and to their managers – and to the potential for conflict between the two systems.

The potential for the third dimension, of broad public accountability to provide a framework for reconciliation between professional and managerial accountability is appealing. Such an idea would be at the heart of the concept of accountability on the grounds of its recourse to 'the people' for arbitration. However, reality is more complex, with at least two broad types of public accountability. First, there is centralized political accountability to central government, secured through the chain of command of general managers who work to a set of objectives shaped largely by national priorities. Second, there is decentralized political accountability; that is, to the people. However, while the NHS increasingly claims sensitivity to 'local voices' (NHSME, 1992), the availability of political sanctions only at a national level is a blunt instrument for ensuring services are appropriate to local needs. Given that local needs may be inconsistent with national priorities, there is an inevitable central–local dilemma for political accountability in the NHS (Hunter, 1992).

Furthermore, 'the public' may be interpreted in a variety of ways within different domains of accountability. For professionals, the public is not perceived as a whole, but as a subset of individual patients or clients. For local purchasers and provider managers, the public comprises a local population whose health needs are to be assessed, service priorities determined and delivered to contract specifications. At the broadest level of public accountability, central Government is responsible for satisfying taxpayers (who are all potential service consumers) regarding the appropriate use of funds for health care. It would seem to follow that the notion of public accountability cannot be applied in a simple way to arbitrate in disputes between professionals and managers.

Accountability and Conflict

Harrison makes the fundamental point that different forms of accountability need not result in conflict, if values are common to all parties (Harrison, 1988b). However, such a consensus seems unlikely. At the heart of disputes between professionals and managers is a basic difference in orientation between, on the one hand, the twin pillars of professional accountability (primacy of the relationship between professional and client, and quality control through peer review) and, on the other hand, cornerstones of managerial accountability (such as the need to adopt a collective, population approach to matters of efficiency and effectiveness, and the belief that managers are responsible for controlling quality). New summarizes this tension, by arguing that the accountability of professionals to their peers is 'insufficient in a publicly funded agency which must be accountable for how limited resources are distributed among competing claims' (New, 1993, p. 128).

The effect of these tensions between professional and managerial approaches are critical in the linked fields of needs assessment and setting priorities, since these decisions shape resource allocation and service delivery. The next section of this chapter explores the shifting territory of accountability for NHS professionals through an examination of needs assessment, and setting priorities for a selected group of health professionals: community health nurses.

Conflict in practice: Community health nursing

Within the NHS, most commentary and analysis on the impact of managerialism on the professions has focused on the most powerful health profession: medicine. However, there are at least two reasons for examining nursing more closely; the first reason is the size of the profession. Numerically, nursing is the largest profession in the NHS: nurses deliver 80 per cent of direct patient care; and their pay accounts for around 25 per cent of all NHS expenditure (NHSE, 1995). If efforts are to be made to improve efficiency and effectiveness, nursing is an obvious choice for increased attention.

A second reason for opting to look at nursing in the context of accountability relationships follows the argument of Day and Klein (1987) that the extreme characteristics of medicine as a profession (such as high social status and esoteric knowledge) can lead to an oversimplification of the accountability debate. Their research suggested that the differential capacity of professionals to make their activities 'invisible' to managers was more critical than simple status in the ability of professionals to define the 'language of evaluation' (Day and Klein, 1987, p. 241).

Taking up this argument in respect to nursing, community health nursing is potentially an illuminating area for study. This 'new and unified discipline' (UKCC, 1994) covers the work of practice nurses (employed by GPs), together with other community-based nurses, such as district nurses; school nurses; occupational health nurses; mental health and mental handicap nurses; children's nurses and health visitors. The work of these nurses is wide-ranging, and spans health promotion, illness prevention and clinical nursing care.

Nurses working in community settings have a higher degree of 'invisibility' (and therefore autonomy) than colleagues in the hospital sector, on two counts. First, on a practical level, managerial supervision is more difficult in community settings, given the peripatetic nature of this nursing work. Second, at a policy level, the work of community-based professionals has traditionally been the subject of comparatively 'little high level policy and management attention' (NHSME, 1993) compared with that in the hospital sector. Accordingly, information systems are poorly developed, adding to the 'invisibility' of community-based work.

However, recent national policy shifts in favour of both community-based care and health promotion have brought increased policy and managerial interest in the work of these nurses (see for example, Department of Health, 1989, 1992). Indeed, according to the (then) NHS Management Executive, community health nursing is now 'at the forefront of a health service revolution' (NHSME, 1993, p. 1).

A description of nursing as a 'profession' is contested, as shown by the debate on the accuracy (and desirability) of this label (see for example, Salvage, 1985; Abbott and Wallace, 1990). It is not the purpose of this chapter to add to this debate, but to view nursing as a 'profession' here on the relatively relaxed criterion that nurses comprise an occupational group with internal systems for accountability, for example, securing standards of practice through training and disciplinary procedures.

Professional accountability in nursing

The United Kingdom Central Council for Nursing, Midwifery and Health Visiting (UKCC) is the regulatory body with responsibility for professional standards and discipline within the profession. Qualified nurses who wish to practice are required to register with the UKCC and to abide by the UKCC Code of Professional Conduct and the Scope of Professional Practice (UKCC, 1992a, 1992b). These documents are couched in terms of the primacy of the relationship between the nurse and the individual patient or client, although they also refer to a wider responsibility to 'serve the interests of society' (UKCC, 1992a). Such normative codes are a somewhat weak device for ensuring professional standards, given their emphasis on the broad values of the profession, rather than on setting and policing standards. In practice, compliance with professional norms has been secured traditionally through a hierarchical system of self-management by the profession.

Peer review is widely regarded as underdeveloped in nursing, and can be a particular problem for community health nurses, working largely in isolation. In common with many other professional bodies, the UKCC has recently developed a quality control system based upon continuing post-qualification development (UKCC, 1994). However, given a profession so large in number, and varied in composition, the content of updating activities is defined only sketchily. While imprecision is no doubt pragmatic, lack of clarity as to what is expected must potentially undermine the scheme in terms of securing acceptable and consistent standards.

Managerial arrangements for community health nurses vary. Practice nurses are employed and managed by GPs. Other community health nurses are employed by a variety of NHS trusts, some of which are dedicated community trusts, others incorporate hospital services. Trust management structures vary considerably, so nurses are managed in different ways. One important trend in the context of accountability has been the removal of an assumption that nurses should be managed by nurses. Managers are increasingly sought for their managerial, rather than professional, skills. This would appear to threaten the capacity of professionals to 'appropriate the currency of accountability' (Day and Klein, 1987, p. 56).

The contested nature of need

It is commonly said in respect of community health nursing services that needs are changing (see for example, Department of Health and Social Security, 1986; Welsh Office, 1987; Royal College of Nursing, 1992), for instance: many traditional threats to public health, by way of epidemics, have been conquered; advances in technology are prolonging the lives of many people with chronic conditions; changes in policy emphasis are designed to facilitate more care in community settings. Yet, it is not just needs themselves that are changing, but also the response of health services. Stewart argues that we have shifted from a position in which service providers recognized needs in a 'uniform' fashion to one in which many perspectives are recognized, leading to 'management of uncertainty' (Stewart, 1990).

Uncertainty derives, in large part, from recognition that the concept of need is contested (Williams, 1974; Bradshaw, 1977; Weale, 1983; Bull, 1990; Doyal and Gough, 1991), not only among and between professionals, but also among and between managers, purchasers and the public. It follows that incorporation of different perspectives in assessing needs and determining priorities is not only a larger task than before, but requires negotiation. In turn, negotiation demonstrates the nature of power relationships between the various 'stakeholders'.

Needs assessment

Since the health reforms of 1991, purchasers have been responsible for identifying and prioritizing the health needs of local populations and for commissioning services to meet these needs by contracting with NHS provider units. This process is informed by the 'epidemiological approach' (Wessex Institute of Public Health Medicine, 1994), which operates at a collective, population-based, level with a focus on disease.

Setting priorities according to a 'population/disease' approach poses two related problems for community health nursing; the *type* and the *level* of needs assessed. First, working at the boundary between health and social care, and attempting to pursue a holistic approach to assessing needs, nurses in community settings are likely to acknowledge needs of a social type, relevant to health, which they could address, but which are outside the remit of health care purchasing.

Second, in terms of the level of assessment, the top-down, population, focus of the epidemiological approach is very different from the bottom-up emphasis of nurses on assessment of the needs of individuals. Discussing the difficulties of using epidemiology as a basis for purchasing, Bull (1990) shows concern with both the type and level of assessment:

> Epidemiology, the science upon which health needs assessment is supposed to be based, is concerned with the levels and distribution of disease in the community ... Each patient, however, is a unique set of social and physical problems which may or may not relate to an identifiable disease.

Setting priorities

The dilemma of 'individual versus collective' focus is central to the question of how the notion of equity is to be interpreted in setting priorities. These two different approaches represent two extremes of view on equity in distribution of resources for health care, which Alwyn Smith (1990, p. 187) summarizes as follows:

> The debate resolves essentially into whether health and medical care should be used primarily to reduce health variance or to increase its mean. Is it to be viewed as contributing to the economic output of the nation or as part of the apparatus of social justice?

While purchasers – and so, through the discipline of contracting, provider managers – are driven by the economic output (or efficiency) approach, the focus of community health nurses on individuals might be interpreted as priority-setting, according to principles of social justice. But what does the latter mean in practice?

Unlike the hospital sector, which uses waiting lists as a means of regulating demand, there is no formal equivalent for community health nursing services. This is not to say that rationing is absent; rather, that the concept has not been applied in policy terms. It falls to professionals to operate a system of rationing based on individual professional judgment. As McIntosh (1993) notes, setting priorities is 'not part of the language of nursing'; rather, rationing procedures used by individual nurses are 'enmeshed in everyday practice'.

Urging nurses to make their priority-setting processes more explicit, McClelland (1993) criticizes 'long standing misapprehensions' held by policy-makers about community health services; that they 'do not have the same demand problem [as hospital services] and thus are instantly available and accessible'. She suggests that at the root of nurses' apparent denial that they set priorities is the sense of inadequacy professionals feel when confronted with needs they do not have time to meet – given doctrines of professional accountability that require all identified health needs of individuals to be met. In practice, she argues, nurses develop and manage personal backlogs – effectively waiting lists – of clients.

The hidden nature of this unmet need is important for two reasons. First, since the criteria for rationing are unclear, such an implicit approach creates difficulties in teasing out how decisions about priorities actually relate to needs (Parker, 1991), with the risk of hidden inequity for individual users (Wilson-Barnett, 1992). Second, needs that are not identified cannot be brought to the attention of managers and purchasers.

Managers, too, face the dilemma of priority-setting at the broad level of resource allocation. In a study of managers' strategies for identifying and dealing with unmet needs for community health nursing, Jacoby (1990, p. 1414) noted that managers were beset by the same problem of the lack of a formal mechanism for regulating demand: '. . . we can't say the beds are full – when do we say enough is enough?'

Jacoby found that, while managers agreed that traditionally nurses had set priorities according to individual professional judgment, managers argued that setting priorities was a managerial task; part of matching resources with activities in a manner designed to optimize value for money. Jacoby (1990) noted several strategies for setting priorities developed by managers, for instance: introduction of waiting lists; targeting activity through tighter eligibility criteria; and closer definition of the role of nursing to eliminate 'social care' activities. These kinds of activities are also reported elsewhere (see for example, NAHAT, 1991; UNISON, 1993).

Nurses themselves do appear to be developing a more explicit approach to setting priorities. For instance, in respect of targeting, health visitors have developed 'at risk' criteria (for example, South East Kent Community Health-care (NHS) Trust, 1991; Walker and Crapper, 1995) and hierarchical categories of need (McClelland, 1993), while much effort within the district nursing service has been expended on the development of dependency measures.

McClelland's push for the concept of 'priority-setting' to be both owned up to and developed by community health nurses, can be seen as part of a wider debate on the distribution of power in resource allocation between managerial and professional values. In this context, nurses are urged to move away from a reactive stance to consider the benefits of a more pro-active approach to meeting needs (Twinn *et al.*, 1990; Wilson-Barnett, 1992). These benefits might be two-fold; first, maintenance by nurses of the power to define their role; and, second, a more pro-active approach is increasingly thought necessary in the quest to demonstrate effectiveness, through illuminating and distinguishing between sound and unsound professional practice (McIntosh, 1993). Certainly, community health nurses – in particular, health visitors – have found problematic the contemporary focus on measurable outcomes, given the preventive nature of much of their work, together with particular difficulties in attributing outcomes directly to their interventions (Lightfoot, 1994).

A shift to managerialism by professionals?

To what extent do these changes in approach by nurses suggest a shift by professionals towards adopting a managerialist perspective? Certainly the drive for proof of effectiveness appears to have stemmed from the rigours of contracting rather than from within the profession itself. But while managers and professionals may agree that setting priorities is an integral part of both an efficient and effective use of resources, *criteria* for setting priorities may still differ between professional and managerialist perspectives.

For instance, while managers commonly wish district nurses to withdraw from providing a bathing service for people whose needs are deemed 'social' rather than 'health' related, some nurses object on the grounds of their holistic definition of health, and the opportunistic assessment of health needs that is possible during bathing activity. This is not to say that nurses do not, in principle, subscribe to a more targeted use of their skills in the context of limited resources; rather, that the means of achieving this are contested. The 'invisibility' of community health nursing exacerbates tension, since neither information on nor conceptual understanding about needs, roles and outcomes in respect of this work is readily available to managers (Lightfoot *et al.*, 1992). As Day and Klein note, information is the 'lifeblood of accountability', and is useless without an 'agreed framework of meaning' (1987, p. 243).

Interestingly, while the traditional strength of nurses in needs assessment is at the level of the individual (Mansfield, 1992; Royal College of Nursing, 1992), there are also now calls – largely from advocates of the 'new public health' movement – for community health nurses to embrace the more collective notion of assessment of the health of the local community (for example, Cernik and Wearne, 1992; Mansfield, 1992; Royal College of Nursing, 1992; Nottingham Community Health NHS Trust, 1993). Such a shift could form an important bridge between the traditional bottom-up, individual focus of nurses, and the top-down, population focus of purchasers and managers responsible for broad resources allocation.

The significant change for nurses in assessing the needs of the community is that an assessment is required of the 'community as client', rather than perceiving the community as the sum of assessments of individual needs (Cernik and Wearne, 1992). Such a change not only arguably requires different skills, but also a sense of an aggregate perspective on needs, which may complement the population-level work of purchasers, which is often broken down into commu-nities, or 'localities'. However, given disparity between nurses and purchasers over the definition of need, closer scrutiny of their respective work on community needs might reveal that here, too, criteria vary in assessment.

Overall, while it appears that professionals may have begun to embrace some tenets of managerialism (perhaps in order to survive in the new system), different perspectives on needs assessment and setting priorities suggest that conflict persists between professionals and managers in terms of a struggle for power to determine the 'language of evaluation'. The final section of this chapter considers how tensions between professionals and managers might be reconciled.

Harmonizing the Domains of Accountability

It is possible to envisage at least two broad options for the future; an adversarial or conciliatory model. Will professionals and managers ultimately pursue an adversarial approach, battling for supremacy? Or might a conciliatory approach develop, with a search for common values?

An adversarial model assumes that the actions of managers will continue to be perceived as an attack on the professions, at least by the latter. On the face of it, managers would appear likely to win such a struggle, since they have both political power (as agents of central Government) and practical power through the control of resources. However, in practice, managers are required to recognize and negotiate in a context of local circumstances, personalities and power (Barrett and McMahon, 1990), in which the activities of professionals are critical in turning policy into practice (Lipsky, 1980; Dalley, 1991). Furthermore, as Harrison and Pollitt suggest in a discussion about rationing, managers – and politicians – may see benefits in professionals retaining a degree of autonomy:

> Such (rationing) decisions are invariably controversial . . . and managers
> are not spectacularly more willing than politicians to take public and
> personal responsibility for unpopular choices. A measure of clinical
> autonomy is therefore protective of managers, as well as of politicians.
> (1994, p. 142)

In practice, professionals and managers depend upon each other for successful service delivery. If, as Day and Klein argue, accountability requires an 'agreed framework of meaning' (1987, p. 243), perhaps an adversarial model should be rejected in favour of an alternative, more conciliatory, approach.

A conciliatory model concerns the prospects for finding a common focus, or common values, between professionals and managers. It might be possible to envisage two broad approaches to conciliation: first, a *radical* approach, in which a different focus is adopted to that normally followed by either professionals or managers; and, alternatively, a *pragmatic* approach might be followed, with emphasis on the management of conflict. Taking the radical approach first, looking beyond disputes between professionals and managers for conciliation recalls a theme explored earlier in this chapter; that is, the prospects for a new emphasis on wider public accountability. If authority is ultimately derived from 'the people', perhaps it is here that binding arbitration can be found. Barbour asserts that 'increased involvement of the public' is the solution to the problem of 'lack of any accepted mechanism for reconciling the allocation of scarce resources with the health care needs and aspirations of society as a whole' (1989, p. 55).

It is not so clear just how such involvement might be best achieved. Central Government has tended to advocate an indirect approach, in which managers and professionals are exhorted to focus more upon users. Examples of this approach include the use of Patient's Charters, and encouraging District Health Authorities to view themselves as consultative 'champions of the people' (NHSME, 1992). However, as a mechanism for public accountability, this approach is weak, since without effective censure by the public, both the agenda for consultation and the extent of subsequent action is still determined by managers and professionals.

Proposals for more effective local public accountability are advanced as a more direct attempt to secure commitment to local communities. How might this be achieved in practice? While recently central Government has proposed delegation of 'accounting officer' status to individual health authority and trust chief executives in a bid to improve local financial accountability (Butler, 1994, p. 6), there have been more radical calls – from both ends of the political spectrum – for greater democratic control of health services through transferring their responsibilities to local Government (for example, see Harrison *et al.*, 1991; Dimbylow, 1993, p. 5).

A more direct means of securing effective public accountability might be participation of the public in the design, delivery and evaluation of health services. According to Pollitt, such an approach would constitute 'a new and highly legitimate source of opinion on "what should be done"' (1993, p. 195). However, Pollitt acknowledges that renewal of traditional ideas about public accountability is perhaps somewhat idealistic today, with few examples to work from in modern, and complex, societies. Certainly, experiments in user involvement in health service rationing decisions have revealed how difficult the notion of such involvement is to put into practice. This is so, not only due to the varying and changing preferences of individuals, and problems of their access to relevant information, but also an expectation of the part of the public that managers and professionals are legitimately charged with decisions about rationing (Heginbotham, 1992).

If a radical focus on public accountability is somewhat idealistic for reconciling tensions between professionals and managers, perhaps the answer lies in more *pragmatic* approaches. Several commentators have stressed the importance of cooperation between professionals and managers. For example, Elston (1991) suggests that cooperation, rather than external forces, is likely to change behaviour, for instance in raising standards. New (1993) talks about the benefits of building a common culture ('normative control') which, as a strategy for securing effective accountability, is both cheap and preventive in terms of avoiding conflict.

There are some suggestions that professionals might be beginning to adopt the ideology of managerialism; for instance, Barbour (1989) refers to a 'new realism' in which professionals take on (and thereby legitimate) managerial initiatives, such as audit. In the case of nursing, King attempts to turn the debate on its head, suggesting that managerial emphasis on setting objectives and evaluating outcomes is usurping the territory of the nursing profession:

> This is nothing new to nurses. The fundamental process of nursing is based on assessing need, setting objectives, planning and delivering care, and reviewing its outcome. (1993, p. 21)

At the heart of conflict between professionals and managers is their difference in focus, the emphasis of the professional is on the individual patient or client and the managers' on a more collective approach. Even here there are signs of a shift by professionals. In the case of community health nursing, making more explicit the existence and process of setting priorities, and embracing a broader 'community as client' approach, are examples of a more collective focus by professionals. Recognition by professionals of a wider 'social responsibility' (Wilding, 1982) offers possibilities for bridging top-down and bottom-up approaches to needs assessment. One practical way forward might be to incorporate more nurses into purchasing teams (Department of Health, 1993).

Given the interdependence in practice between professionals and managers, Scrivens (1988) highlights the importance of searching for mechanisms through which managers might recognize and harness the contribution which profession-als can make to meeting organizational objectives. In the case of 'invisible' community health nurses, such mechanisms might include: using knowledge gained through local needs profiling activities; and using the experience of professionals to define appropriate data for information systems (King, 1993). The appropriateness of incorporating professional advice in meeting the objectives of health authorities, is recognized by Government in its proposal to make such advice a legislative requirement (NHSE, 1995).

Since managers cannot control professional accountability – but never-theless require assurance of its effectiveness – enlightened managers might seek to strengthen processes of professional accountability, rather than attempt to supplant them with managerial approaches. For example, Harrison (1988b) suggests that managers might improve in-house opportunities for developing peer review. They might also recognize and build upon existing professional quality assurance initiatives (Pollitt, 1990).

Increased openness about priority-setting by nurses not only makes their process of professional accountability more explicit but, in identifying for managers and purchasers the nature and extent of unmet needs, it also reinforces the dividing line between professional and managerial accountability. Whilst making unmet needs explicit does not ensure that they are subsequently met, professionals can redefine the problem as managerial rather than professional in character.

Overall, this final set of ideas for strengthening professional accountability and harnessing its results possibly represents the most realistic way forward in the short term. But Pollitt (1990) notes that matters cannot be left to professionals alone. Also needed are both the political spur which comes from the active involvement of users and the organizational push which comes from the systematic analytical skills of managers, both of which are arguably as yet underdeveloped. In other words, we cannot escape the need for a better understanding of the relationship between professional, managerial and wider public accountability.

Conclusion

There can be no doubt that accountability is a complex issue. While this chapter has attempted to sketch out some of the territory to be addressed, there are many avenues to be explored in more detail. Such exploration requires empirical investigation in order to tease out the meaning of accountability in its practical context. We might expect the balance of influence between professional, managerial and public accountability to vary according to factors such as: the degree of 'invisibility' of the profession; the capacity of managers to impose an alternative vision; and the scope for local people (including service users) to express their views. One potentially fruitful area for analysis might be to examine how tensions between professional and managerial accountability are reconciled by first line managers with a professional background.

What is clear is that growing policy attention is focused on accountability in the health care system, and that the existence of several types of accountability is formally recognized. For example, the NHSE is publishing guidance on the accountability of GP fundholders in response to widespread concerns about the scope of their autonomy. The guidance identifies four types of accountability applicable to GP fundholding: management; financial; professional; and accountability to patients and the wider public (NHSE, 1994). However, the potential conflicts between these elements are not identified.

This chapter has argued for the accountability of professionals to be incorporated more explicitly into debates about accountability – debates that have traditionally been dominated by the analysis of the relationship between political and managerial accountability. The argument for bringing professional accountability into sharper focus rests upon the traditional autonomy of welfare professionals and challenges to this position of power by, largely, a new managerialist ideology.

The ultimate question must be whether users are better served by a professional or managerial emphasis. For this reason, a more systematic incorporation of user and public voices in policy and practice might mediate between professional and managerial approaches, based upon principles of public accountability. While such mediation might be a long term prospect, an important preliminary step would be commitment by both managers and professionals to make *explicit* the bases of their judgments, so that the nature and scope of their decisions can be open to scrutiny.

References

ABBOTT, P. and WALLACE, C. (1990) 'The sociology of caring professions: an introduction', in ABBOTT, P. and WALLACE, C. (Eds) *The Sociology of Caring Professions*, London: The Falmer Press.

BARBOUR, J. (1989) *Notions of 'Success' in General Management*, Health Services Management Research, **2**(1), pp. 53–7.

BARRETT, S. and McMAHON, L. (1990) 'Public management in uncertainty: a micro-political perspective of the National Health Service', *Policy and Politics*, **18**(4), pp. 257–68.

BRADSHAW, J. (1977) 'The concept of social need', in FITZGERALD, M.R., HALMOS, P., MUNCIE, J. and ZELDIN, D. (Eds) *Welfare in Action*, London: Routledge and Kegan Paul.

BULL, A.R. (1990) 'Perspectives on the assessment of need', *Journal of Public Health Medicine*, **12**(3/4), pp. 205–8.

BUTLER, P. (1994) 'Plan to boost NHS accountability is widely welcomed', *The Health Service Journal*, **104**(5388), pp. 6.

CERNIK, K. and WEARNE, M. (1992) 'Using community health profiles to improve service provision', *Health Visitor*, **65**(10), pp. 343–5.

DALLEY, G. (1991) 'Beliefs and behaviour: professionals and the policy process', *Journal of Ageing Studies*, **5**(2), pp. 163–80.

DAY, P. and KLEIN, R. (1987) *Accountabilities: Five Public Services*, London: Tavistock.

DEPARTMENT OF HEALTH (1989) *Caring for People: Community Care in the Next Decade and Beyond*, Cm 849, London: HMSO.

DEPARTMENT OF HEALTH (1992) *The Health of the Nation: A Strategy for Health in England*, Cm 1986, London: HMSO.

DEPARTMENT OF HEALTH (1993) *A Vision for the Future: The Nursing, Midwifery and Health Visiting Contribution to Health and Health Care*, London: DH.

DEPARTMENT OF HEALTH AND SOCIAL SECURITY (1983) *National Health Service Management Enquiry*, HC (84) 13 (Chair: Roy Griffiths), London: DHSS.

DEPARTMENT OF HEALTH AND SOCIAL SECURITY (1986) *Neighbourhood Nursing – A Focus for Care. Report of the Community Nursing Review* (Chair: Julia Cumberlege), London: HMSO.

DIMBYLOW, E. (1993) 'Wandsworth seeks control of local health services', *Public Finance*, 12 November, p. 5.

DOYAL, L. and GOUGH, I. (1991) *A Theory of Human Need*, London: Macmillan.

ELSTON, M.A. (1991) 'The politics of professional power: Medicine in a changing health service', in GABE, J., CAENAN, M. and BURY, M. (Eds) *The Sociology of the Health Service*, London: Routledge.

HARRISON, S. (1988a) 'The workforce and the new managerialism', in MAXWELL, R. (Ed.) *Reshaping the National Health Service*, Oxford: Transaction Books.

HARRISON, S. (1988b) *Managing the NHS: Shifting the Frontier?* London: Chapman and Hall.

HARRISON, S., HUNTER, D.J., JOHNSTON, I., NICHOLSON, N., THUNHURST, C. and WISTOW, G. (1991) *Health Before Health Care*, London: Institute for Public Policy Research.

HARRISON, S., HUNTER, D.J., MARNOCH, G. and POLLITT, C. (1989) 'General management and medical autonomy in the National Health Service', *Health Services Management Research*, **2**(1), pp. 38–46.

HARRISON, S. and POLLITT, C. (1994) *Controlling Health Professionals*, Buckingham: Open University Press.

HEGINBOTHAM, C. (1992) 'Rationing', *British Medical Journal*, **304**, pp. 496–9.

HUGMAN, R. (1991) *Power in Caring Professions*, London: Macmillan.

HUNTER, D.J. (1992) Accountability and the NHS, *British Medical Journal*, **304**, pp. 436–8.

JACOBY, A. (1990) 'Management strategies and patient needs: the provision of nursing care in the community', *Journal of Advanced Nursing*, **15**, pp. 1409–17.

JENKINS, K., CAINES, K. and JACKSON, A. (1988) *Improving Management in Government: The Next Steps*, London: HMSO.

JOHNSON, N. (1974) 'Defining accountability', *Public Administration Bulletin*, **17**, December, pp. 3–13.

KING, W. (1993) *Defining the Data*, Primary Health Care, **10**(3), pp. 21–2.

LEVITT, R. and WALL, A. (1992) *The Reorganised National Health Service*, 4th Edn, London: Chapman and Hall.

LIGHTFOOT, J. (1994) 'Demonstrating the value of health visiting', *Health Visitor*, **67**(1), pp. 19–20.

LIGHTFOOT, J., BALDWIN, S. and WRIGHT, K. (1992) *Nursing by Numbers? Setting Staffing Levels for District Nursing and Health Services*, York: Social Policy Research Unit, University of York.

LIPSKY, M. (1980) *Street-level Bureaucracy: Dilemmas of the Individual in Public Service*, New York: Russell Sage Foundation.

McCLELLAND, A. (1993) 'Community nurse waiting lists', letter in *Health Visitor*, **66**(1), p. 34.

McINTOSH, J. (1993) *Assessment and Prioritising of Need for Nursing Care in the Community*, paper for Queen's Nursing Institute Conference 'Nursing in Europe: Common Problems, Common Solutions', May.

MANSFIELD, J. (1992) *Key Issues in District Nursing Paper Three: Challenges for District Nursing*, London: District Nursing Association UK.

NAHAT (NATIONAL ASSOCIATION OF HEALTH AUTHORITIES AND TRUSTS) (1991) *Care in the Community: Definitions of Health and Social Care – Developing an Approach. A West Midlands Study*, Research Paper No 5, Birmingham: NAHAT.

NEW, B. (1993) *Accountability and Control in the NHS*, Health Care UK 1992/3, pp. 117–35, Newbury: Policy Journals.

NHSME (NHS MANAGEMENT EXECUTIVE) (1991) *Resource Management in the Community Health Services*, London: DH.

NHSME (NHS MANAGEMENT EXECUTIVE) (1992) *Local Voices: The Views of Local People in Purchasing for Health*, London: DH.

NHSME (NHS MANAGEMENT EXECUTIVE) (1993) *New World, New Opportunities: Nursing in Primary Health Care*, London: HMSO.

NHSE (NHS EXECUTIVE) (1994) *An Accountability Framework for GP Fundholding: Towards a primary care-led NHS*, (for consultation), Leeds: NHSE.

NHSE (NHS EXECUTIVE) (1995) *Professional Involvement in HA Work*, EL(95)61, Leeds: NHSE.

NOTTINGHAM COMMUNITY HEALTH NHS TRUST (1993) *The Public Health Post at Strelley: An Interim Report*, Nottingham: Nottingham Community Health NHS Trust.

PARKER, J. (1991) *Priority Families – How Are They Defined by Health Visitors?* Bristol: Avon College of Health.

PETERS, B.G. (1989) *The Politics of Bureaucracy*, 3rd Edn, New York: Longman.

POLLITT, C. (1990) 'Doing business in the temple? Managers and quality assurance in the public services', *Public Administration*, **68**, Winter, pp. 435–52.

POLLITT, C. (1993) *Managerialism and the Public Services*, 2nd Edn, Oxford: Blackwell.

ROYAL COLLEGE OF NURSING (1992) *A Powerhouse for Change: Report of the Taskforce on Community Nursing*, London: RCN.

SALVAGE, J. (1985) *The Politics of Nursing*, London: Heinemann.

SCRIVENS, E. (1988) 'The management of clinicians in the National Health Service', *Social Policy and Administration*, **22**(1), pp. 22–34.

SMITH, A. (1990) 'The ethics of resource allocation: symposium proceedings', *Journal* of Epidemiology and Public Health, **44**, pp. 187–90.

SOUTH EAST KENT COMMUNITY HEALTHCARE (NHS) TRUST (1991) *Matching Resources to Need: Reprofiling*, Community Nursing Service, Folkestone: SE Kent Community Healthcare (NHS) Trust.

STEWART, J. (1990) 'Meeting needs in the 1990s' in CALLAGHAN, B., COOTE, A., HOLME, G. and STEWART, J. (Eds) *Social Policy Paper No 2*, London: Institute for Public Policy Research.

TWINN, S., DANNCEY, J. and CARNELL, J. (1990) *The Process of Health Profiling*, London: HVA.

UKCC (UNITED KINGDOM CENTRAL COUNCIL FOR NURSING, MIDWIFERY AND HEALTH VISITING) (1992a) *Code of Professional Conduct*, London: UKCC.

UKCC (UNITED KINGDOM CENTRAL COUNCIL FOR NURSING, MIDWIFERY AND HEALTH VISITING) (1992b) *The Scope of Professional Practice*, London: UKCC.

UKCC (UNITED KINGDOM CENTRAL COUNCIL FOR NURSING, MIDWIFERY AND HEALTH VISITING) (1994) *The Future of Professional Practice – the Council's Standards for Education and Practice Following Registration*, London: UKCC.

UNISON (1993) *Bringing It All Home*, London: UNISON.

WALKER, M. and CRAPPER, E. (1995) 'Identifying families of concern', *Primary Health Care*, **15**(2), pp. 12–14.

WEALE, A. (1983) *Political Theory and Social Policy*, London: Macmillan.

WELSH OFFICE (1987) *Nursing in the Community – A Team Approach for Wales* (Chair: Noreen Edwards), Cardiff: Welsh Office.

WESSEX INSTITUTE OF PUBLIC HEALTH MEDICINE (1994) *Health Care Needs Assessment: The Epidemiologically Based Needs Assessment Reviews*, Oxford: Radcliffe Medical Press.

WILDING, P. (1982) *Professional Power and Social Welfare*, London: Routledge and Kegan Paul.

WILLIAMS, A. (1974) '"Need" as a demand concept (with special reference to health)', in CULYER, A.J. (Ed.) *Economic Politics and Social Goals: Aspects of Public Choice*, York Studies in Economics, London: Martin Robertson.

WILSON-BARNETT, J. (1992) 'Priorities in allocating nursing resources', *Journal of Advanced Nursing*, **17**, pp. 645–6.

Chapter 10

Social Policy in a Multi-Racial Britain: The Case of Community Care

Karl Atkin

Social policy's neglect of 'race' is deeply rooted. The discipline's origins, grounded in Fabian ideals, emphasize the politics of collectivism, and the practice of state intervention to deal with social problems (Pinker, 1971). This Fabian approach assumes commonly agreed policy objectives, but fails to recognize the needs of different social groups. Further, in dealing with social problems, it emphasizes the principles of organization and administration and confines analysis to discrete policy areas such as education, health and employment (Williams, 1989). Conceptual cleavages, such as class, race, disability and gender are ignored (Williams, 1989; Squires, 1990). More specifically the ideas of early Fabianism were also marked by racial bigotry and superiority, by a belief in a hierarchy of 'races' and by a nationalist programme of social imperialism (Williams, 1996). For example, founders of the Fabian movement – such as George Bernard Shaw, Beatrice and Sydney Webb – were all members of the Eugenics movement.[1] The national and racialist assumptions implicit in the work of the earlier Fabians re-emerged as the discipline of social policy, and informed the development of the post-war welfare state. Internationally, it assumed the civilizing mission of imperialism and 'the duty to help and guide the teeming millions of India and Africa to a more abundant life' (Titmuss, 1943, p. 9). In terms of the nation state, the discipline of social policy maintained pride in Britain and the British welfare state. The 1942 Beveridge report, for example, uncritically accepted the importance of maintaining the British race and values.

Massive immigration during the 1950s and 60s did little to alter these assumptions. Black and Asian people were invited to Britain to solve labour shortages and ensure the continued growth of the British economy. Yet the potential impact of mass immigration on welfare provision was ignored by Government policy (Cashmore and Troyna, 1990). Indeed their solution to the problem – evident in a series of immigration acts – was to reduce the number of New Commonwealth migrants entering, or having the potential to enter, the UK. Other potential solutions, such as improving the conditions in which black and ethnic minorities lived, and tackling the racism experienced by them, were not considered. Social policy uncritically accepted theories of assimilation, and the idea that people from black and ethnic minorities would soon conform to the established cultural norms of the 'host' society, thereby disappearing as an identifiable group of people. In one of the earliest Fabian discussions surrounding race, a pamphlet examining the impact of mass immigration on education policy argued: 'immigrants ... must not only be taught English, they must also be taught about Britain. Their lack is not merely words but of the feel for situations which native speakers of the language have' (Deakin and Lester, 1967). The 'assimilation' approach to race relations, and the assumption that the unrestricted entry of black and Asian people had caused social problems went largely unquestioned by social policy. Consequently inequality and disadvantage, supposedly central themes of social policy analysis, were not applied to the experiences of black and Asian people.

During the 1970s and 80s, there were sustained theoretical challenges to mainstream thinking, resulting in the gradual breakdown of Fabian theoretical dominance (Taylor-Gooby, 1985; Williams, 1989). There is no doubt that some social policy commentators are slowly responding to the significance of 'race' (cf. Barham *et al.*, 1992; Blakemore and Boneham, 1995). For example, Fiona Williams (1989), by challenging mainstream thinking, has provided an outline of how social policy has marginalized 'race': in terms of its failure to acknowledge the experience and struggles of black people; and account for racism in the provision of welfare services. However, despite the valuable insights offered by writers such as Fiona Williams, 'race' is still rarely afforded systematic treatment in most mainstream social policy research. If mentioned at all, the subject is regarded as a specialist area, having little relevance to mainstream social policy; or is subsumed under general problems such as 'poverty' or the 'inner city' (cf. Bean and MacPherson, 1983; Glennerster, 1983). More specifically, there is little evidence that mainstream social policy has become informed by the more theoretical critiques of multiculturalism or the development of anti-racist methodologies (cf. Jones, 1991). Further empirical research – central to the Fabian ideal of using evidence to inform social change – has largely failed to reflect challenges to mainstream thinking. Social policy research, by default, has focused almost exclusively on the white populations of the UK (Atkin, 1991).

The neglect of black and ethnic minorities by social policy analysis mirrors their neglect by successive Governments' policies. Nonetheless, just as social policy is slowly coming to terms with a multiracial Britain, Government policy guidance on issues such as housing, health and social care are beginning to mention the specific 'linguistic and cultural needs' of ethnic minorities. Recent policy debates on community care, for example, are beginning to acknowledge the multiracial nature of British society (cf. Department of Health, 1989). This chapter, by examining community care policy and its impact on black and Asian people, attempts to illustrate the more general problems facing social policy analysis. By using community care as a case study, it demonstrates the importance of 'race' for the discipline of social policy and introduces conceptual tools designed to understand the experience of black and Asian people, as well as attempting to account for the racism they experience. In particular, the conceptual tools emerging from this specific case study can be applied to other areas of social policy: employment, housing and education, thus enabling a full account of welfare provision that includes the experience of black and ethnic minorities.

Community Care in a Multi-racial Britain

Recent debates on community care have begun to recognize the 'particular care needs' of Britain's ethnic minority populations (cf. Department of Health, 1990; Audit Commission, 1992). Specifically, 'good community care' must recognize the 'circumstances of minority communities', be sensitive to their needs, and be planned in consultation with them (cf. Department of Health, 1989). Recognition of the 'particular care needs' of minority groups at the 'highest level of policy making' has been described 'as something of a breakthrough' (Walker and Ahmad, 1994). More significantly, this recognition occurs as health and social services are undergoing the most substantial changes since the beginning of the post-war state (Wistow *et al.*, 1994). Bureaucratic and paternalistic forms of public services have been undermined, and new means of achieving allocation, delivery and production have been sought (Hambleton, 1988). Although precise definitions remain contested, ideals such as citizenship, consumerism, participation, and choice have emerged as key policy objectives in attempting to empower recipients of community care services. The restructuring of community care is the product of two specific concerns. First, in common with most European countries, the UK Government is facing increasing expenditure on welfare provision, and is under pressure to control public spending. Using existing budgets more efficiently to achieve more appropriate targeting of resources emerges as a central aspect of Government policy (cf. Audit Commission, 1986). Second, and as a reaction to the long struggle to offer dignity to disabled and older people, Government policy has questioned the responsiveness of community care services. Griffiths' (1988) agenda for action on community care, for example, argued that community service delivery was poorly related to need. This echoed the concerns of an earlier Audit Commission report that emphasized the importance of 'a flexible service response' that offered a wider range of options (Audit Commission, 1986).

Government policy presents 'markets' as the most effective panacea to the difficulties described above. Specifically, the idea that market efficacy, rather than collective planning mechanisms, is the best way of ensuring efficiency, accountability and choice in community care, is at the heart of Government health and social care policy. To achieve this, the 1990 NHS and Community Care Act introduced the separation of purchasing and providing functions in public health and social care agencies (Enthoven, 1985). Notions such as the 'internal market' and 'the mixed economy' of care form the organizational basis from which to provide community care services. The general principles informing the restructuring of community care provide the overall framework in which the rhetoric of 'good community care' for black and ethnic minorities will be realized. The specific consequences of this restructuring for black and ethnic minorities are discussed later in the chapter. The introduction of the new community care, however, does not exist in a vacuum and changes cannot be discussed without reference to the existing disadvantages facing people from ethnic minorities.

Community care and institutional racism

Empirical evidence suggests that community care provision experiences considerable difficulties in recognizing, and responding to, the needs of people from black and ethnic minorities (Dominelli, 1989; Atkin and Rollings, 1993; Walker and Ahmad, 1994; Butt, 1994). Black and Asian users often characterize community service provision as being difficult to communicate with, slow to respond, narrow in perspective, resistant to pressure and unwilling to understand. Problems of access to, and appropriateness of, community health and social services have been well established. Conceptually, *institutional racism* emerges as fundamental in explaining this inappropriate and inaccessible provision.

Institutional racism occurs when the policies of an institution lead to racially discriminatory outcomes for users of minority ethnic communities, irrespective of the motives of individual employees in the institution (Cashmore and Troyna, 1990). More specifically, institutional racism has been described as camouflaged (Glasgow, 1980), meaning it is not open or particularly visible, and is embedded in the taken for granted assumptions informing organization practices. Further examination of institutional racism suggests two key issues emerge: structural barriers to service delivery; and the neglect and misrepresentation of the needs of black and ethnic minorities.

Structural barriers and racism

Welfare provision's inability to recognize the structural barriers to provision facing black and Asian people represents a fundamental form of institutional racism. This is manifest in assumptions such as *same service to all*, which irrespective of needs, equates with *equal service to all*. Consequently services are organized according to a 'white-norm' and do not recognize difference and diversity; assuming their policies, procedures and practices are equally appropriate for everyone (Atkin and Rollings, 1993; Blakemore and Boneham, 1995). Straightforward examples include the inability of health and social services to provide support for people who do not speak English, or more specifically the unavailability of vegetarian food or halal meat in day care and domiciliary services. Such practices legitimate non-recognition of the community care needs of minority ethnic communities and disregard the dietary, linguistic and caring needs of minority ethnic communities.

Further, assuming everyone has equal access to services privileges the white population by ignoring the obstacles faced by black and Asian people in gaining access to services (National Association for Health Authorities, 1988). Black and Asian people do not have the same opportunities as the white population; they experience greater disadvantage and suffer more barriers to service receipt (Glendinning and Pearson, 1988). Racial inequalities and poverty disadvantage black and Asian people and create additional needs for support. Providing an equal service for all ignores the consequences of this. Evidence on racial inequalities in income, employment and housing is overwhelming (Skellington and Morris, 1992). Although far from homogenous, the average income of Asian (particularly Pakistani and Bangladeshi) and Afro-Caribbean families living in the UK is well below that of 'white' families, and unemployment rates among black and ethnic minorities are about twice the national average. Further, within the Pakistani and Bangladeshi communities there is relatively little participation of women in the labour market, thus affecting family income and access to contributory benefits. For a variety of reasons, Asian and black families are also less likely to receive their full social security entitlements (Gordon and Newham, 1985; Law, 1993). Housing, another important factor in community care, suggests further inequalities. Minority ethnic communities are more likely to be in older, un-modernized, inner-city housing, which is damp and draughty, as well as lacking central heating and other household amenities such as washing machines (Skellington and Morris, 1992). Asian and Afro-Caribbean families also carry a disproportionate burden of homelessness. The experience of older people provides a specific example of the structural disadvantage facing people from ethnic minorities. Most old people, be they black or white, face similar patterns of disadvantage including poor housing, poverty, low income, and social isolation. Older black people, however, are further disadvantaged. As a consequence of recent arrival they are often ineligible for full state pensions and few have occupational pensions. Their incomes, therefore, are likely to be lower than those of older white people (Norman, 1985). Evidence also suggests that older black and Asian people experience greater social isolation; many older Asian people, for example, cannot speak English and may be afraid to leave their homes because of the possibilities of racist attacks.

Misrepresentation of health and social care needs of minority ethnic groups

The second manifestation of institutional racism is the misrepresentation of the needs of black and ethnic minorities. In particular, health and social services often identify black health and social 'problems' as arising from cultural practices. This approach, and the criticism of it, has significance not only for community services but also for present debates about ethnicity, race and social policy. Therefore it is worthwhile examining the various strands of this debate and its implications for tackling institutional racism. Much of the policy debate on race and community care in explaining differences between the majority white population and minority black population, conceptualizes the issue in terms of cultural pluralism and ethnic diversity (Lawrence, 1982; Atkin, 1991). This approach has become known as multiculturalism, and finds expression in other policy areas such as education (Rattansi, 1992). According to multicultural approaches, diversity in language, religion, cultural norms and expectations prevent effective communication, and create misunderstanding between the majority and distinct minorities. Overcoming the linguistic and cultural barriers that cause misunderstandings and promoting awareness of the other's culture should result in more sensitive and responsive services.

There are several problems with this view, notably the relationship between ethnically distinct minorities and the majority white society is seen exclusively in terms of cultural practices (Gilroy, 1982). Within this largely uncritical framework, the outcome is to present 'white' culture as the norm. This diverts attention from the wider power relationships within society, and in particular fails to recognize that the dominant white culture and the distinct minority culture do not meet on equal terms. The situation of black people cannot be solely understood in terms of cultural artifacts – the political, social and economic positions of black people are equally important. As we have seen, black and Asian people experience many barriers to welfare provision as a consequence of structural disadvantage, but a narrow account of culture does not accommodate this structural dimension.

Despite these criticisms, the emphasis on culture is evident in the response of health and social services. To accommodate 'cultural difference', health and social services often establish 'specialist provision'. The idea of 'special provision' in welfare services has a long history, and represents the most popular means by which mainstream services feel they are implementing equal opportunity policies (Butt, 1994). However, the existence of 'special provision', although often beneficial in responding to the needs of black and Asian communities, does not necessarily imply that their needs are being adequately met (Patel, 1990). Separate provision, for instance, is too often a euphemism for short-term, inadequately funded and marginal provision (Patel, 1990; Butt, 1994). Further, mainstream services often use the existence of specialist services to absolve themselves of any responsibility for the health, and social care needs of black and ethnic minorities. By pointing to this 'special provision', statutory provision has remained relatively static and inaccessible (Ahmad and Atkin, 1996 forthcoming). Establishing 'special provision' has led to internal divisions within minority ethnic communities, with groups competing with each other on the basis of 'culturally distinctive needs'. More conceptually, the use of the term 'special' to describe provision to black and Asian people infers their needs are somewhat unusual (Atkin and Rollings, 1993). Black and Asian people, although sometimes having different needs from the majority white population, do not necessarily have 'special needs'. To consider they do, implies that black and Asian minorities' 'distinctiveness' is a 'problem' requiring a 'special' response. Such classification segregates black and Asian people from the general debate about social care, isolating them from the mainstream discussion.

The emphasis on cultural practices also has more pernicious consequences, potentially resulting in service organizations 'blaming' the potential client group. Black and ethnic minorities are either blamed for experiencing specific problems or censured for failing to understand an organization's aims. For example, black and Asian people are frequently characterized as in some way to blame for their own needs because of deviant and unsatisfactory lifestyles (Cameron *et al.*, 1989). There is a history of defining health problems faced by minority ethnic communities in terms of cultural deficits, where a shift towards a 'western' lifestyle is offered as the main solution to their problems. Rocherson (1988), for example, argues that the Asian Mother and Baby Campaign, organized by the Health Education Authority to encourage greater use of post-natal services, defined the need of Asian women in a way that defends, rather than questions dominant professional practices. The problems associated with Asian women's care are restricted to cultural aspects, and the campaign makes no reference to the structural disadvantage associated with race, gender or class. More recently, disability among Asian communities has been attributed to diet and consanguineous marriages. Ahmad (1995) has argued that this approach reflects yet another example of racism masquerading as medical science. Further, the preoccupation with cultural practices in explaining disability ignores other explanations – such as the role of poverty in causing ill-health (Atkin, 1991).

Cultural stereotypes and myths

As a consequence of multiculturalism, minority ethnic groups have to contend with inappropriate generalizations of cultural practices, and the use of simplistic socio-cultural explanations to understand their behaviour. Introductory notes on black communities, present in most training material for service practitioners, often follow this pattern. One would not, for instance, attempt to summarize a western approach to child rearing practices in one paragraph, yet this is what black people are subject to (Durrant, 1989). A text on community nursing further demonstrates the shortcomings of this approach (Karseras and Hopkins, 1987). The authors suggest that, although health professionals dislike 'being authoritarian' and aim for 'reasoned persuasion', Asian women do prefer 'a blunter response' and are 'not offended by imperatives'. Generally, neat cultural packages identifying key characteristics of black people do not solve the problems facing community care services, and are likely to perpetrate and reinforce cultural stereotypes and myths.

A particularly spurious myth, evident in the activities of community care services, is the assumption that Asian people, and to a lesser extent Afro-Caribbean people, live in self-supporting families. This is often used as an excuse for not making necessary changes to the existing services, or expanding the level of service provision to meet the needs of black and ethnic minorities (Atkin and Rollings, 1993; Walker and Ahmad, 1994). This is despite substantial evidence suggesting this view of the extended family is unjustified because it does not take into account the process of immigration, as well as ignoring the diversity among black and ethnic minority groups. The extended Afro-Caribbean family has always been rare in the UK, and a third of Afro-Caribbean people live alone (Baxter, 1988). Further, a survey in Leicester suggests that 40 per cent of Afro-Caribbean people do not have frequent family contact (Farrah, 1986). Consequently, many Afro-Caribbean people are not only isolated in a household sense, but do not have frequent family support (Eribo, 1991). Although the extended family is common among Asian families (Barker, 1984) there are still a significant proportion of Asian people who live alone with few relatives in this country (Fenton, 1987). In addition, economic and demographic factors – such as appropriate housing and occupation mobility – may influence the willingness and ability of Asian families to provide care, thus making the extended family less prevalent (Owen, 1993). There is already considerable variation between the generally larger Bangladeshi and Pakistani households, and the smaller Sikh and Hindu households (Owen, 1993). This is accompanied by challenges to marriage patterns, both internally and by immigration rules (Fenton, 1987). Brah (1978) noted that by the late 1970s Asian adolescents were expressing some unease with traditional marriage customs, many looking forward to forming a 'nuclear' household, while keeping in close contact with the 'joint family'. Restrictive immigration policies also leave families divided (Fenton, 1987). More importantly, however, it is questionable whether living in an extended family should be used as a justification for not providing service support. The general belief that the extended family has the material and emotional resources to meet the needs of family members can lead to neglect by default (Atkin and Rollings, 1993).

The role of culture?

Not surprisingly, the general emphasis on cultural practices among welfare services to explain the behaviour of Asian and black people has been subject to extensive criticism (Gilroy, 1982). Consequently 'anti-racist' approaches, emphasizing the importance of structural disadvantage in understanding the experience of black and Asian people, have emerged. In examining structural disadvantage, anti-racist approaches have tended to dismiss cultural descriptions as a surrogate form of racism. For reasons outlined above, this has led to a perhaps understandable distrust of cultural descriptions. On the other hand, it is impossible to ignore the importance of 'culture' and 'identity' in understanding the experience of people from black and ethnic minorities (Stuart, 1993). Black people are more than a product of the racism they experience.

The conceptualization of 'culture' by multicultural approaches is the problem rather than the concept of 'culture' *per se*. Particularly since multi-cultural approaches tend to strip culture of its dynamic social, economic and gender context (Ahmad, 1995). Consequently 'culture' becomes a rigid and constraining concept, mechanically determining people's behaviour and actions. As we have seen, 'neat cultural packages' perpetuate rather than challenge myths and stereotypes. Black and Asian cultures are not static, unitary or monolithic, but as complex as white culture. Cultural generalizations, encouraged by multi-cultural approaches, fail to recognize that culture is a creative resource, combining spatial and temporal components (Bourdieu, 1977). Culture provides a flexible resource for living, and ascribing meaning to one's feelings and experience. Cultural norms provide guidelines for understanding and action that predispose individuals to certain types of response. They do not, however, determine that response. Cultural norms are open to different interpretations between people and over time, and are structured by social cleavages; previous experience; relationships; resources; and priorities. For examples, descriptions of Hindu, Sikh or Muslim behaviour often transpose the situation in Asia to Britain, ignoring the process of migration. The emergence of a 'Black British' population will subtly remould the 'traditional' cultural norms of their community. Black and Asian people need to reconcile two or more cultural backgrounds, thus establishing a creative tension. Cultural ties with their place of origin may still be strong yet they are faced with situations where they have to accommodate western ways and values. They have anchorage in two or more distinct cultures, but do not fully belong to either. For black and Asian people living in Britain it is not a matter of forsaking one culture for another but finding the space to express both.

To be successful and overcome the impact of institutional racism, policy and practice has to become informed by black people's own perceptions of care in the community, and this means an understanding of people's culture. Cultural differences do generate misunderstandings, but perceptions of culture should not become identified as 'inferior' and 'deviant'. Difference is not a problem in itself. The notion of 'otherness' does not address the extent to which the taken for granted norms of the white majority are equally socially constructed. It is not that black minorities are culturally different; rather that we are all different culturally (Ballard, 1989). This approach has to understand these differences in the context of the political, social and economic disadvantage faced by black and ethnic minorities, and in particular the racism they experience.

Racist attitudes and service providers

Before leaving this discussion of racism, reference should be made to the potential effect of racist attitudes held by frontline practitioners. These attitudes can deprive minority ethnic communities of their rights to services, especially since health and social service professionals exercise considerable discretion in their day-to-day work (Lipsky, 1980). Racist attitudes, however, are not distinct from institutional forms of racism. Often, for example, the values and assumptions of service practitioners represent an expression of institutional forms of racism and it is difficult to disentangle the two. Further, accounts that emphasize examples of individual racism can be criticized for misunderstanding and simplifying the operation of racism. For instance, if the problems facing black and ethnic minorities are considered a consequence of racist attitudes, the solution is to offer training that challenges these attitudes. It is possible, therefore, to 'cure' racism. This approach, however, ignores the embedded nature of racism in the institutional practices of British society, and the structural disadvantage facing Britain's black and ethnic minorities.

Nonetheless, racist attitudes on the part of service practitioners have been reported in a number of studies of health and social services (Foster, 1988; Ahmad *et al.*, 1989; Cameron *et al.*, 1989; Bowler, 1993), and have led to black and Asian people being denied access to service provision. For example, practitioners working in local authorities often list black people as 'high risk' clients, 'uncooperative' and 'difficult to work with' (Cameron *et al.*, 1989; Dominelli, 1989; Atkin and Rollings, 1993). Similarly, evidence suggests that racism within the NHS affects virtually all black people with common stereotypes, portraying black people as 'calling out doctors unnecessarily', 'being trivial complainers', and 'time wasters' (Glendinning and Pearson, 1988; Ahmad *et al.*, 1989). More specifically, Badger *et al.* (1988) suggested that district nurses tend to assume homogeneity among their black and Asian clients, and explained behaviour in terms of simplistic cultural stereotypes. Foster (1988) identified similar racist attitudes among health visitors. Comments made by health visitors included the view that minority groups should give up their culture, and conform to the norms of British society, and that black patients were a problem.

The New Community Care

The existing disadvantages facing people from black and ethnic minorities and the consequences of institutional racism provide the context in which the current restructuring of health and social care is introduced. How then do the solutions offered by the NHS and Community Care Act relate to the problems faced by black and ethnic minorities? Perhaps not surprisingly, evidence suggests there remains widespread uncertainty, puzzlement and ignorance about what should be done to meet the needs of black and Asian minorities among health and social services (Butt, 1994; Walker and Ahmad, 1994). Policy remains undeveloped and rarely goes beyond bland statements supporting the principles of racial equality, while the mechanisms that might achieve race equality, and the principles that underlie them remain unexplored.

Initially, it is questionable whether devices such as the internal market, the separation of purchaser and provider roles, the mixed economy of care and the enabling role of social services can deal with the fundamental disadvantage faced by black and ethnic minorities. Choice does not necessarily follow from 'market' competition. Market principles on their own, without a wider commitment to tackling racism, do not challenge the racist assumptions, stereotypes and myths evident in the activities of practitioners, purchasers, planners and policy makers. If anything, the institutional nature of racism means that market principles may end up compounding the disadvantages faced by black and ethnic minorities. Indeed evidence suggests allocative decisions are likely to reflect the inequalities that exist in society and therefore perpetuate the structural disadvantage faced by certain social groups (Papadakis and Taylor-Gooby, 1987). Three specific practical examples originating from the restructuring of community care services further demonstrate some of the potential problems facing black and ethnic minorities.

First, when drawing up contract specification and service level agreements, purchasers should ideally commit the provider agency to racial equality and equal opportunity, and ensure the agency provides evidence proving their competence to provide services effectively (Rooney and McKain, 1990). Evidence suggests, however, that health and social service departments, although able to introduce contract specifications to ensure equal opportunities and equitable service provision, do not have either the ability or resources to enforce them (Walker and Ahmad, 1994). Moreover, devolving responsibility for equal opportunities policy to individual organizations creates an additional problem of maintaining a coherent and sustainable commitment to such a policy (Atkin, 1995). The difficulty of maintaining equitable service delivery would seem to rest with individual providers rather than as a more general problem facing welfare provision. Decisions about allocations that disadvantage black and Asian people become obscured, and are seen as a consequence of an individual rather than a collective response. Responsibility for disadvantage becomes diffuse and fragmented thus making racism all the more difficult to tackle. The general effect of institutional racism is ignored, and is replaced by an account that explains racism in terms of the dysfunction of individual organizations.

Second, increased efficiency may be obtained at the expense of accessibility and quality . Much of the time in drawing up contract specification is spent on ensuring social service departments can measure success or failure, rather than on deciding what success or failure mean (Butt, 1994). This emphasis could potentially mean 'success' being measured in financial terms rather than terms of the quality of service being provided. Moreover, the pressures on local authorities and health authorities to achieve low unit cost could force them into block contracts with large scale service providers offering a standardized service, insensitive to the needs of black and Asian people.

Third, the mixed economy of care increases the importance of voluntary sector provision (Atkin, 1995). Mainstream voluntary sector provision, however, experiences similar problems of ethnocentric and discriminatory service provision to those of health and social services (Field and Jackson, 1989). Norman (1985), for instance, describes 'a long established voluntary sector' that has done little to recognize that we live in a multiracial society – whether in employment policy; staff and volunteer training; committee membership; relationships with ethnic minority voluntary organizations; or provision of services to individuals in minority groups. Other research suggests these voluntary organizations seem unclear about what an equal opportunities policy is, and many have no awareness of the detailed monitoring and follow-up procedures such policies would involve (Dungate, 1984). Not surprisingly, low take-up of voluntary sector services by black and Asian minorities is common, despite a demonstrated demand for these services (Field and Jackson, 1989). Black and Asian voluntary provision, which offers a solution to inaccessible and inappropriate service delivery, is under-developed and underresourced (Jeyasingham, 1992). The enabling and mobilizing role the NHS and Community Care Act gives to social services is unlikely to rectify these problems. The assumptions and practices that deny black and Asian users access to appropriate services outlined above are likely to persist in this enabling role (Atkin, 1995).[2] As we have seen, statutory services are described as narrow in perspective, and unwilling to understand the difficulties faced by black voluntary sector providers. Further, local authorities' preference for consulting and negotiating with well established, professional, predominantly white voluntary sector organizations compounds the problem (Walker and Ahmad, 1994). Black and Asian voluntary sector providers therefore are ill-equipped to offer competition (Jeyasingham, 1992) as they negotiate more barriers with fewer resources (Walker and Ahmad, 1994).

The future development of community care

Health and social service provision has not been responsive to the views of people from black and ethnic minorities. The current restructuring of community care services, seems unlikely to change this as the reforms do not tackle the embedded disadvantage faced by black and ethnic minorities. This failure, however, is not an inevitable consequence of a mixed economy of care. Levick (1992), for example, castigates 'counsels of despair' and argues that legislation is made up of contradictory and changeable elements that create the alternative of 'radical possibilities'. A similar belief is held by Harrison (1993), who argues policy analysis needs to acknowledge the struggles black people engage in.

More generally, writings on 'race' and social care tend to focus on the problems of accessibility and appropriateness, as well as general disadvantage in the provision of services (Atkin and Rollings, 1993). The evaluation offered by this chapter draws on such material, and highlights the unfair structuring of opportunities. The critical emphasis of the literature on 'race' and social care is perhaps understandable, and has successfully highlighted the negative consequences of racism, marginalization and unequal treatment. By focusing on disadvantage there is a danger, however, of adopting a 'victim oriented' perspective. This victim oriented approach advocates a paternalist solution to the problems faced by black and Asian people while neglecting the possibility of empowerment. Moreover, by highlighting the negative consequences of service provision there is a danger that this does little to advance thinking and practice (Levick, 1992).

Government policy on health and social care has dangers as well as opportunities. It simultaneously raises the possibility that needs of minorities may be swept aside and marginalized, while also presenting the opportunity of needs-led care planning, the opening of consultation and planning processes to direct local influence, a new awareness of carer's needs, and a recognition of the particular circumstances of black and ethnic minorities (Walker and Ahmad, 1994). These opportunities arise in the context of existing demands, and in particular the challenges of providing appropriate community care services to black and Asian communities (Butt, 1994; Walker and Ahmad, 1994). Black and Asian minorities, as we have seen, do not enjoy equality of access to social and health services, and the current changes in community care do little to alter that.

Conclusion

The central concerns of social policy such as social security, the personal social services, the health service, education, employment and housing are subject to extensive research activity. Yet challenging questions regarding a multiracial society are still largely ignored. This chapter, by using community care as a case study, describes and accounts for racism in the provision of welfare services. It introduces theoretical debates able to inform social policy analysis. Conceptual tools, such as institutional racism are relevant to all aspects of welfare provision, and are not specific to community care services.

Straightforward examples from housing provision, employment and education illustrate this. The embedded practices of local authority housing departments, for example, have been shown to disadvantage black and ethnic minorities (Skellington and Morris, 1992). Common assumptions include the view that black people are 'better off' living in areas with other black people, rather than living in white-dominated suburbs. Such policies result in people from black and ethnic minorities being placed in inner city areas that are often characterized by a shortage of resources and facilities (Cashmore and Troyna, 1990). This perpetuates the disadvantages faced by black and ethnic minorities. Further, TUC analysis of unemployment figures show that black and Asian people are seven times more likely to lose their jobs than white people (Trade Union Congress, 1994). Discrimination in hiring and firing practices was identified as the main cause of unemployment amongst black workers. The average unemployment rate for black workers increased from 11 per cent to 17 per cent between 1990 and 1992, but for white workers the increase was 6 per cent to 9 per cent. Finally, education provides many examples of institutional racism: there is considerable evidence, for example, that demonstrates a systematic tendency for able black students to be allocated to sets and streams and entered for examinations below their capabilities (Rattansi, 1992). Careers advice given to both Afro-Caribbean and Asian children is frequently based on conceptions of their supposedly unrealistic and overambitious aspirations. Attempts are then made to route black children into low-level manual work, regardless of ability or level of motivation. On a more practical level, various institutional practices work against black and Asian students (Rattansi, 1992). Rules about appropriate forms of dress provide one example. Schools, for example, have been known not to allow Sikh boys to wear turbans or girls to cover their legs. Other instances include a lack of availability of vegetarian food or halal meat; the failure to communicate school messages to parents in languages other than English; and the absence of policies on racial abuse or equal opportunities.

Race, rather than a marginal concern, is of fundamental importance to social policy, and needs to be incorporated into mainstream social policy thinking. The present restructuring of welfare provision, however, creates a potential obstacle to this. These changes represent the most fundamental rethink of welfare provision since the Beveridge report, but there is a danger that the discipline of social policy will revert back to its traditional focus of concern – the organization and delivery of services. This would lock social policy into an analysis that continued to neglect social cleavages such as race, gender and social class. Yet as we have seen, the introduction of quasi-markets is not independent of the existing disadvantage facing black and ethnic minorities. Social policy must attempt to integrate an account of race and ethnicity in all policy work, otherwise it will fail in one of its fundamental aims – to offer a complete analysis of welfare provision.

Notes

1　Other members of the Eugenics movement included social reformers such as the Cadburys, John Keynes and William Beveridge.
2　Under the NHS and Community Care Act, Social Service Departments were allocated the strategic tasks of mobilizing new sources of care, and coordinating their delivery. In this respect, they are to become *enabling* authorities that make 'maximum possible use of private and voluntary providers' (Department of Health, 1989).

References

AHMAD, W.I.U. (1995) 'Reflections on the consanguinity and birth outcome debate', *Journal of Public Health Medicine*, **16**(4), pp. 423–8.

AHMAD, W.I.U. and ATKIN, K. (1996 forthcoming) 'Caring for a disabled child: The case of children and sickle cell or thalassaemia', *British Journal of Social Work*.

AHMAD, W.I.U., KERNOHAN, E.E.M. and BAKER, M.R. (1989) 'Health of British Asians: A research review', *Community Medicine*, **11**, pp. 49–56.

ATKIN, K. (1991) 'Health, illness, disability and black minorities: A speculative critique of present day discourse', *Disability, Handicap and Society*, **6**(1), pp. 37–47.

ATKIN, K. (1995) 'An opportunity for change: Voluntary sector provision in a mixed economy of care', in ATKIN, K. and AHMAD, W.I.U. (Eds) *Race and Community Care*, Buckingham: Open University Press.

ATKIN, K. and ROLLINGS, J. (1993) *Community Care in a Multi-Racial Britain: A Critical Review*, London: HMSO.

AUDIT COMMISSION (1986) *Making a Reality of Community Care*, London: HMSO.

AUDIT COMMISSION (1992) *Community Care: Managing the Cascade of Change*, London: HMSO.

BADGER, F., CAMERON, E. and GRIFFITHS, R. (1988) 'Put race on the agenda', *The Health Service Journal*, **98**(5129), pp. 1426–7.

BALLARD, R. (1989) 'Social work with Black people: What's the difference', in ROJECK, C., PEACOCK, G. and COLLINS, S. (Eds) *The Haunts of Misery: Critical Essays in Social Work and Helping*, London: Routledge.

BARHAM, P., RATTANSI, A. and SHELLINGTON, R. (1992) *Race and Anti-Racism*, London: Sage.

BARKER, J. (1984) *Black and Asian Old People in Britain*, Mitcham: Age Concern.

BAXTER, C. (1988) 'Black carers in focus', *Cancerlink*, **4**, pp. 4–5.

BEAN, P. and MACPHERSON, S. (1983) *Approaches to Welfare*, London: Routledge and Kegan Paul.

BEVERIDGE, W. (1942) *Social Insurance and Allied Services*, Cmnd 6404, London: HMSO.

BLAKEMORE, K. and BONEHAM, M. (1995) *Age, Race and Ethnicity*, Buckingham: Open University Press.

BOURDIEU, P. (1977) *Outline of a Theory of Practice*, Cambridge: Cambridge University Press.

BOWLER, I. (1993) 'They're not the same as us: Midwive's stereotypes of South Asian maternity patients', *Sociology of Health and Illness*, **15**, pp. 157–78.

BRAH, A. (1978) 'South Asian teenagers in Southall: their perceptions of marriage, family and ethnic identity', *New Community*, **6**(3), pp. 197–206.

BUTT, J. (1994) *Same Service or Equal Service?* London: HMSO.

CAMERON, E., BADGER, F., EVERS, H. and ATKIN, K. (1989) 'Black old women and health carers', in JEFFERYS, M. (Ed.) *Growing Old in the Twentieth Century*, London: Routledge.

CASHMORE, E. and TROYNA, B. (1990) *Introduction to Race Relations*, London: The Falmer Press.

DEAKIN, N. and LESTER, A. (1967) *Policies for Equality, Fabian Research Series 626*, London: The Fabian Society.

DEPARTMENT OF HEALTH (1989) *Caring for People: Community Care in the Next Decade and Beyond*, Cm 849, London: HMSO.

DEPARTMENT OF HEALTH (1990) *Community Care in the Next Decade and Beyond: Policy Guidance*, London: HMSO.

DOMINELLI, L. (1989) 'An uncaring profession? An examination of racism in social work', *New Community*, **15**(3), pp. 391–403.

DUNGATE, M. (1984) *A Multiracial Society, The Role of National Voluntary Organisations*, London: Bedford Square Press.

DURRANT, J. (1989) 'Moving forward in a multiracial society', *Community Care*, **792**, pp. iii–iv.

ENTHOVEN, A.C. (1985) *Reflections on Management of the National Health Services*, London: Nuffield Provincial Hospital Trust.

ERIBO, L. (1991) *The Support You Need: Information for Carers of Afro-Caribbean Elderly People*, London: Bedford Square Press.

FARRAH, M. (1986) 'Black elders in Leicester: an action research report on the needs of Black elderly people of African descent from the Caribbean', *Social Services Research*, **1**, pp. 47–9.

FENTON, S. (1987) *Ageing Minorities: Black People as They Grow Old in Britain*, London: Commission for Racial Equality.

FIELD, S. and JACKSON, H. (1989) *Race Community Groups and Service Delivery*, London: HMSO.

FOSTER, M.C. (1988) 'Health visitors' perspective on working in a multi-ethnic society', *Health Visitor*, **61**, pp. 275–8.

GILROY, P. (1982) 'Steppin' out of Babylon: race, class and autonomy', in Centre for Contemporary Cultural Studies, *The Empire Strikes Back*, London: Hutchinson.

GLASGOW, D. (1980) *The Black Underclass*, New York: Jossey Bass.

GLENDINNING, F. and PEARSON, M. (1988) *The Black and Ethnic Minority Elders in Britain Health Needs and Access to Services*, Health Education Authority in Association with the Centre for Social Gerontology, University of Keele.

GLENNERSTER, H. (1983) *The Future of the Welfare State*, London: Heinemann.

GORDON, P. and NEWHAM, A. (1985) *Passport to Benefits*, London: Child Poverty Action Group.

GRIFFITHS, R. (1988) *Community Care: An Agenda for Action*, London: HMSO.

HAMBLETON, R. (1988) 'Consumerism, decentralisation and local democracy', *Public Administration*, **66**, pp. 125–47.

HARRISON, M. (1993) 'The black voluntary housing movement: Pioneering pluralistic social policy in a difficult climate', *Critical Social Policy*, **13**(3), pp. 21–35.

JEYASINGHAM, M. (1992) 'Acting for health: Ethnic minorities and the community health movement', in AHMAD, W.I.U. (Ed.) *The Politics of Race and Health*, Bradford: Race Relations Research Unit, Bradford University.

JONES, K. (1991) *The Making of Social Policy in Britain*, London: Athlone.

KARSERAS, P. and HOPKINS, E. (1987) *British Asians: Health in the Community*, Chichester: John Wiley.

LAW, I. (1993) *Racial Equality and Social Security Service Delivery*, Leeds: School of Sociology and Social Policy, University of Leeds.

LAWRENCE, E. (1982) 'In the abundance of water the fool is thirsty: Sociology and Black pathology', in Centre for Contemporary Cultural Studies, *The Empire Strikes Back*, London: Hutchinson.

LEVICK, P. (1992) 'The janus face of community care legislation: An opportunity for radical possibilities?' *Critical Social Policy* **12**(1), pp. 75–92.

LIPSKY, M. (1980) *Street-level Bureaucracy: Dilemmas of the Individual in Public Service*, New York: Russell Sage Foundation.

NATIONAL ASSOCIATION FOR HEALTH AUTHORITIES (1988) *Action Not Words: A Strategy to Improve Health Services for Black and Ethnic Minority Groups*, London: National Association of Health Authorities.

NORMAN, A. (1985) *Triple Jeopardy: Growing Old in a Second Homeland*, Policy Studies in Ageing, 3, London: Centre for Policy on Ageing.

OWEN, D. (1993) *Ethnic Minorities in Britain (Census Papers)*, Warwick University: Centre for Research in Ethnic Relations.

PAPADAKIS, E. and TAYLOR-GOOBY, P. (1987) 'Consumer attitudes and participation in state welfare', *Political Studies*, **XXXV**, pp. 467–81.

PATEL, N. (1990) *A Race Against Time, Social Services Provision to Black Elders*, London: Runnymede Trust.

PINKER, R. (1971) *Social Theory and Social Policy*, London: Heinemann.

RATTANSI, A. (1992) 'Changing the subject? Racism, culture and education', in DONALD, J. and RATTANSI, A. (Eds) *Race, Culture and Difference*, London: Sage.

ROCHERSON, Y. (1988) 'The Asian Mother and Baby Campaign: The construction of ethnic minorities' health needs', *Critical Social Policy*, **22**, pp. 4–23.

ROONEY, B. and MCKAIN, J. (1990) *Voluntary Health Organisations and the Black Community in Liverpool*, Report of a survey by health and race project, Liverpool: Sociology Department, Liverpool University.

SKELLINGTON, R. and MORRIS, P. (1992) *Race in Britain Today*, London: Sage.

SQUIRES, P. (1990) *Anti-Social Policy*, Brighton: Harvester Wheatsheaf.

STUART, O. (1993) 'Double oppression', in SWAIN, J., FINKLESTEIN, V., FRENCH, S. and OLIVER, M. (Eds) *Disabling Barriers; Enabling Environments*, London: Sage.

TAYLOR-GOOBY, P. (1985) *Public Opinion, Ideology and State Welfare*, London: Routledge and Kegan Paul.

TITMUSS, R. (1943) *Problems of Population*, London: English University Press.

TRADE UNION CONGRESS (1994) *Black Workers in the Labour Market*, London: TUC.

WALKER, R. and AHMAD, W.I.U. (1994) 'Windows of opportunity in rotting frames: care providers' perspectives on community care and Black communities', *Critical Social Policy*, **40**, pp. 46–9.

WILLIAMS, F. (1989) *Social Policy: A Critical Introduction*, Cambridge: Polity Press.

WILLIAMS, F. (1996) 'Race, Welfare and Community Care: An historical perspective', in AHMAD, W.I.U. and ATKIN, K. (Eds) *Race and Community Care*, Buckingham: Open University Press.

WISTOW, M., KNAPP, M., HARDY, B. and ALLEN, C. (1994) *Social Care in a Mixed Economy*, Buckingham: Open University Press.

Chapter 11

The Prospects for Social Policy in the European Union[1]

John Ditch

Introduction

This chapter will consider four themes. First, it will trace the recent development of European social policy, from its inception as a minor component of the founding treaties of the European Community, to its position at the heart of debates about the future of the Union. Second, there will be reflection on the prospects for the convergence or divergence of social policy in terms of policy inputs, outputs and outcomes. Third, there will be a review of the key recommendations of recent EU policy documents, including the Union White Papers on Growth, Competitiveness, Employment and Social Policy. The chapter will conclude by arguing that the substantive (as opposed to rhetorical) distance between the United Kingdom and other member states of the Union is less than is often supposed, and that efforts should be made to reintegrate Britain into the mainstream of EU social policy.

Social policy has never been at the heart of the European Union's strategy. At one level this is surprising, because the founding treaties – their guiding spirits and apostles alike – have been dedicated to the improvement of living and working conditions within each member state. The juridical base for European social policy has always been weak, but under the leadership of Jacques Delors the European Commission was able to pursue a more widely based strategy during the latter half of the 1980s. A high water mark was achieved in the early 1990s, but there was a cost. The United Kingdom Government, long suspicious of what they regarded as unnecessary and counter-productive intervention by the European Community in social policy matters, opted out of the Fundamental Charter (December 1989) and then opted out of the social policy provisions on the Union Treaty signed at Maastricht in 1991.

Against this background, it may seem easy to be pessimistic about the prospects for the European social dimension; certainly there are few grounds for confident optimism. However, the European Commission remains active in the social field, and a brace of White Papers on economic and social policies (CEC 1993, 1994a), coupled with a Medium Term Social Action Programme (CEC, 1995) have established an agenda for future intervention. After a period of uncertainty, and no little confusion about the practical and legal implications of the British opt-out from the social provisions of Maastricht, there is a new confidence that the other (now 14 member states) can move forward under the terms of the Social Policy Agreement without the UK.

Diversity and dissonance within the Union there may be, but equally there is evidence of similar experiences and trends: convergent demographic trends and economic profiles are contributing to growing individualism; more privatization programmes; less social solidarity; greater interest in the environment; a pervasive interest in policy efficiency and effectiveness. At the same time, the rising significance of the principle and practice of subsidiarity are mediating the policy process in ways that make it difficult to assess the extent to which there is either convergence or divergence in policy aims and outcomes.

The Promise of Convergence

Over the past 40 years, there has been recurrent uncertainty about the wisdom and feasibility of achieving the convergence of policy goals and instruments. The ideas that inform the concept of convergence and the factors which inhibit or promote its achievement will be considered in this next section. In the beginning, it was the goal of harmonization, heralded in the Treaty of Rome in 1957, which was the preferred objective. However, this has been displaced in the lexicon of integration strategies by the promise, if not the immediate prospect, of convergence. Harmonization, as originally formulated, was not only an impossible goal to attain but as the Community has developed so its attraction to politicians and public has appeared to diminish. The idea of harmonization was suggestive of sameness and federalism, apparently ascribing to the European Commission a central role in prescribing not only standards to be achieved, but the methods to attain them. Convergence on the other hand, was considered to be less prescriptive and threatening to national interests. It was thought to describe some inexorable trends in wider economic processes and demographic patterns, or to suggest that national policies could be refocused to promote mutually advantageous policy goals. This interest in convergence presupposed a shared vision of the benefits, which might be achieved by a further 'deepening and strengthening' of the Community, and a tolerance of the coordination of policies that such a strategy might imply.

The mission to achieve a Single Europe, devoid of unnecessary barriers to the movement of people, goods and capital, became the primary thrust of

European strategy in the 1980s. An unexpected and somewhat bizarre *pas de deux* between Jacques Delors (the typical European and socialist) and Margaret Thatcher (free marketeer and arch Euro-sceptic) allowed the Single European Act to become a shared reality; but each saw within it a vision of their own making. Whereas Margaret Thatcher saw an open market full of producers, customers and opportunities for trade, Jacques Delors saw a social Europe, a place for citizens living and working in solidarity. The inevitable tension between these two visions has provided the dynamo for both the grand politics of Europe, and the micro politics of social policy for the past decade.

Both visions of Europe were rooted in a theory of convergence. Regrettably they derived from contrasting sides of the Janus construct. Thatcher saw convergence of economies as a natural stage in the development of economic systems; only a little encouragement was required to enable the beneficial consequences to be realized. Delors, on the other hand, while recognizing the power of forces leading to convergence of structures and systems, also saw their capacity to generate division, exclusion and inequality. For him, intervention was necessary not to liberate potential, but to manage dislocation and diswelfare. Each approach can be traced to a theoretical bedrock in post-war social science.

Theories seeking to explain trends towards convergence began to proliferate at the same time as the foundation stones for the new institutions of continental Europe were being laid. The fundamental assumption was that welfare states were a form of economy and polity common to many countries, and which reflected the development of industrial capitalism. The most influential theories laid emphasis on technological determinism as the driving force for social and economic change. The logic and imperatives of industrialism, were considered to subordinate social, political and cultural diversity in pursuit of increasingly similar social structures. Two schools of thought can be identified: firstl, the industrial convergence theory argued that the diversity of pre-industrial society becomes subordinated to occupational segregation, with the inevitable dominance of the 'economic' over the 'social'. In this context, it is a relationship to the labour market that critically determines life chances and, arguably, family forms. A second school of thought, a later variant of the first theory, advanced ideas about the goal of post-industrialism and its correlates (service industries, information technology and professional knowledge) displacing manufacturing and industrial production. Both schools of thought were usually presented in an optimistic and benign manner, affecting to believe that history was unfolding to a secure and harmonious future.

If some theorists argued that similarity and sameness were the by-product of technological change and economic growth, others argued that industrial society actually promoted pluralism and segmentation, thereby diminishing the influence of ideology, and breaking down traditional links between employment, social class, status and power. As societies become more complex and heterogeneous, so traditional loyalties, relationships and communities begin to fragment.

The political as well as theoretical implications of this formulation are important but complex. Both left and right, in Britain and throughout Europe, are aware of the underlying logic: economies are becoming interdependent, more international and dominated by the exigencies of finance capital rather than manufacturing or extraction industries. How the consequences of this process are viewed and responded to, is however, contradictory. In the United Kingdom, and for the past decade or more, a rather simplistic left–right bifurcation has tended to shape the perceptions of advantage and disadvantage in relation to the developing Single Market. The right is seen to be the pro-market but anti-social dimension; the left is seen to be in favour of the social dimension and resigned to the Single Market. In reality the application of this curiously British prism to the dynamics of market and social policy will prove to be too simple. There can be no simplistic division between left and right, between pro and anti European stance.

In summary, three factors need to be taken into account when considering convergence. First, there needs to be clarity about the differences between convergence of inputs, policy instruments, outputs and outcomes. It is conceivable to have convergence of one without convergence of any of the others. Second, it is necessary to take account of time: it is easier to identify indicators of change over a 40 year period than over a 40 month period. Finally, convergence is both an analytic and descriptive category which can be used to report trends but it is also, and importantly in the context of European integration, a political value. Individuals and governments differ over whether and to what extent, convergence of economies or social structures should be regarded as a 'good thing'.

To what extent have the economies and social structures of Europe been moving together over the past 40 years? If they have, can anyone say whether this process has been helped or hindered by the intervention of politicians? There are many weaknesses in the capacity of social scientists to map important distinctions between the convergence or divergence (over time) of policy inputs, outputs and outcomes. In part, this may be because it is notoriously difficult (but probably necessary) for politicians and policymakers to be less than explicit about the precise nature of policy objectives.

Data Sources

In pursuit of clarity, the European Union invests significantly in the collation of statistical data that reports on key indicators of social and economic well-being in Europe. Eurostat, based in Luxembourg, is a clearing house for statistical information. Although it is heavily dependent on the good will and resources (both financial and professional) of the national statistical offices, Eurostat provides a comprehensive, and improving, picture of trends and prospects through a wide array of statistical sources and series. The Single European Act, and the processes which were thereby accelerated, necessitated an enhancement in monitoring capacity. Increasingly there are formal exchanges of data between the major international agencies with the aim of mapping trends in the convergence or divergence of economies, demographies and social structures. However, all is not as well as would be hoped for. In the absence of specific reference points or targets, it becomes increasingly difficult to identify the scope and scale of resource inputs. Leaving to one side the imprecision that complicates, if not confounds measures of GDP, or even population size, there is frequent uncertainty in the purpose of policy intervention: to err may be human but to be ambiguous is the art of a successful policymaker. Allowing for a spurious capacity to quantify/specify indicators of policy input there is greater difficulty when it comes to specifying output. Take for example employment and unemployment.

Comprehensive, reliable, accurate and uncontested data on the labour market are difficult to obtain. Definitions vary between one country and another; they vary, as in the United Kingdom, from one year to another. For example, there are currently about 18 million people unemployed in EU, but in 1992 over 22 per cent of those counted as unemployed using the European Labour Force Survey were not registered as being unemployed by the relevant national authorities; at the same time only 63 per cent of those included in the national figures corresponded to the international definition. The growth in atypical forms of employment, increased numbers of discouraged workers, and economically inactive women mean that the differences are getting wider and not narrower, and this makes for greater difficulty in monitoring and policymaking (CEC, 1994b; ILO World Report, 1995).

Indicators of Convergence

Of much greater interest to citizens and social scientists alike are the outcomes to be achieved in terms of overall living standards or life chances. In this context, and even within a national context, the specification and elaboration of indicators is weak. What is meant by the term quality of life and how can it be measured? Are the indicators to be aggregate or individual, objective or subjective? What account is to be taken, or can be taken, of differences in national context? Against this background of uncertainty there must be caution about quantitative evidence reporting convergence and divergence of outcomes. That said, poor quantitative indicators (and they can be no more) are better than no indicators at all.

Attempts to measure the quality of life in comparative studies are of relatively recent origin. In part this is because the term 'quality of life' means different things to different people: as Scanlon (1993) has put it, the concept 'suffers from an embarrassing richness of possibilities'. As the European institutions have developed, and there has been a rise in levels of material prosperity, there appears to have been a shift away from a preoccupation with meeting material and security needs – in favour of a more general concern with non-material needs, environmental issues and the quality of personal relationships. Inglehart (1990), on the basis of secondary analysis of Eurobarometer data, has styled this movement as being a transition from materialist to post-materialist values. Broadly similar attitudinal structures can be found across national boundaries. Two distinct trends are worth noting however. First, there are significant differences between younger and older cohorts, with the former being more inclined to post-materialist values: these are in the ascendency as the population of Europe ages. Second, there is a curious disjuncture between rising levels of material prosperity (indicated by, for example, measures of GDP per capita) on the one hand, and indicators of subjective well-being on the other. As increased levels of aggregate wealth become translated into increased life expectancy and rising levels of income, there is the possibility that this becomes associated with an emergent gap between aspirations and fulfilment. This is what Inglehart and Rabier (1986) call 'happiness over the next hill'.

Common Problems and Trends

Across Europe there is evidence of common trends and shared problems. For example, there is growing recognition of the impact of demographic change on the demand for services, and the capacity of countries (and individuals) to pay for them.

The primary cause of demographic ageing is the increase in the average life span and in life expectancy at adult ages (see Tables 11.1 and 11.2). These are a product of the impact of medical developments, which in Europe have seen an end of deaths due to infectious diseases, and changes in lifestyle and advances in the treatment of degenerative diseases. In the years immediately preceding the Second World War, life expectancy at birth differed by 10 years between the best and the worst member states: it was just over 50 years for women in Spain, Greece and Portugal, compared with 60 years in Denmark and the Netherlands. The southern countries have more than made up the difference. In the course of 60 years, Spanish women have gained a further 30 years life expectancy (CEC, 1994c).

These demographic trends are stimulating the consideration of a number of common policy options: adjustments to the age at which pensions are paid; the equalization of pension ages; the tightening of eligibility criteria, and a changing balance in the relationship between statutory and supplementary provision; the development of insurance and equity release schemes to meet the costs of long-term nursing and residential care.

Table 11.1: Percentage of population aged 65 and over in 1990 and projections to 2000 and 2020

	1990	*2000*	*2020*
Belgium	14	15	18
Denmark	15	15	20
France	14	15	19
Germany	16	17	22
Greece	12	15	18
Ireland	11	11	13
Italy	14	15	19
Luxembourg	16	16	21
Netherlands	13	14	19
Portugal	12	14	14
Spain	13	14	17
UK	15	14	16
EC (12)	14	15	19

Source: Organization for Economic Co-operation and Development (OECD) (1994) *New Orientations for Social Policy*, Paris OECD, p. 72

Table 11.2: Life expectancy at birth in the year 2020 according to different forecasts in a selection of Member States

	United Nations (1994)		*Eurostat (high scenario)*		*Eurostat (low scenario)*		*Caselli and Egidi (1991)*		*National statistical institutes*	
	M	F	M	F	M	F	M	F	M	F
Denmark	75.5	81.2	77.5	82.0	72.5	78.0	74.6	80.2	72.2	77.7
France	76.9	83.6	78.0	84.5	73.5	81.5	75.7	85.4	78.0	86.5
Italy	78.5	84.3	79.0	84.0	74.5	81.0	78.1	84.5	–	–
Netherlands	77.6	83.2	78.5	83.5	74.0	80.5	77.0	87.2	76.0	81.5
Portugal	75.5	82.0	77.5	82.5	72.5	79.0	76.4	82.6	–	–

Source: CEC (Commission of the European Communities) (1995)

These convergent tendencies are to be placed in the context of common problems and challenges across the EU. For example, and this is a theme that has been adopted in the 1994 EU White Paper on Social Policy, there is a need to establish both an equitable and an efficient relationship between social protection

Table 11.3: Sources of contributions to social protection expenditure as a percentage of total funding – 1990

	Employers' contributions	*Protection persons' contributions*
Belgium	45	27
Denmark	8	5
France	52	29
Germany	41	30
Greece	49	24
Ireland	25	15
Italy	53	15
Luxembourg	31	22
Netherlands	20	39
Portugal	45	21
Spain	55	17
UK	27	15
EC (12)	42	24

Source: CEC (1994d), p. 83

and economic activity. This concern is high on the policy agenda because a lower proportion of the population in EU countries is engaged in gainful employment than in the USA, Japan or the major European Free Trade Association competitor countries (CEC, 1994b). In turn, this relates to the financial structure of social protection (see Table 11.3); the differential impact on wage costs; and the net effect on employment structures and levels.

Inputs

Indicators of convergence have historically concentrated on measures of input or effort. Comparisons of this kind provide a significant opportunity to compare the composition and aggregate volume of expenditure on social programmes over time. A key measure is the proportion of GDP committed to social expenditure (see Table 11.4). For example, we find that the 'golden age' of the international welfare state was in the 1960s and 1970s; this was when spending on social expenditure rose markedly. In 1960 an Organization for Economic Cooperation and Development (OECD) average of 12.3 per cent of GDP was committed to social expenditure; by 1985 this had increased to 24.6 per cent. But the late 1980s saw consolidation if not retrenchment. Over the past 25 years there has been significant narrowing of differences in levels of social expenditure between

Table 11.4: Current social protection expenditure as percentage of GDP, 1970–1991

	B	DK	D	GR	E	F	IRL	I	L	NL	P	UK	EUR (12)
Total social expenditure													
1970	18.7	19.6	21.5	na	na	19.2	13.2	17.4	15.9	20.8	na	15.9	na
1975	24.2	25.8	29.7	na	na	22.9	19.7	22.6	22.4	26.7	na	20.1	na
1980	28.0	28.7	28.7	12.2	18.1	25.4	21.6	19.4	26.5	30.8	14.7	21.5	24.4
1983	30.8	30.1	28.2	17.2	19.5	28.3	24.1	22.9	27.2	33.2	16.1	23.9	25.3
1986	29.4	26.7	28.1	19.4	19.5	28.5	24.1	22.4	24.8	30.9	16.3	24.3	26.0
1989	26.7	29.8	27.5	20.7	20.1	27.6	20.2	23.1	25.2	31.0	16.6	21.9	25.2
1991	26.7	29.8	26.6	na	21.4	28.7	21.3	24.4	27.5	32.4	19.4	24.7	26.0
Social expenditure excluding unemployment compensation													
1970	18.2	19.2	21.3	na	na	19.0	09.4	17.4	15.9	20.2	na	12.5	na
1975	22.7	23.6	28.7	na	na	22.2	17.8	22.2	22.4	25.2	na	19.1	na
1980	25.6	25.7	27.9	11.9	15.4	24.3	20.1	19.0	26.1	28.2	14.3	19.9	23.1
1983	27.5	26.1	27.1	16.8	16.5	27.0	21.1	21.2	27.3	29.1	15.9	21.6	24.5
1986	26.5	24.1	26.8	19.0	16.3	27.1	20.9	21.8	24.6	27.7	15.9	22.3	24.3
1989	24.3	26.7	26.3	20.4	17.1	26.1	17.7	23.1	25.1	28.3	16.3	21.1	23.8
1991	24.6	26.3	25.7	na	17.7	27.0	18.6	24.0	27.2	29.9	19.0	23.6	24.6

Source: CEC (1994d), p. 42

F.11.1

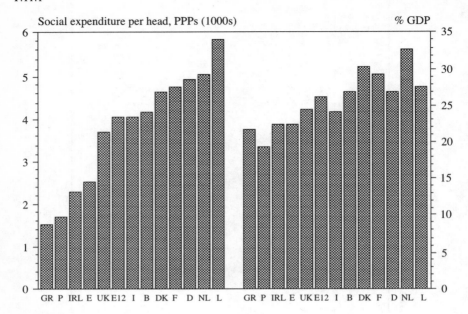

Figure 11.1: CEC (1994d), p. 41

EU Member States. From relatively low levels, spending has increased in the southern countries, while spending in the northern countries has stabilized.

For the Union as a whole, expenditure on social protection amounted to 26 per cent of total GDP. In other words almost 4000 ECU (about £3280 stg) was spent per person. But this average marks a wide range (see Figure 11.1).

It is apparent that expenditure varies, in general terms, with levels of economic prosperity. Expenditure is highest in those countries with high levels of incomes per head – Netherlands (32.4 per cent), Denmark (29.8 per cent). In 1991, the UK committed 24.7 per cent of GDP, which was just below the EC average. On a per capita basis (and using purchasing power parities) the highest level of expenditure is to be found in Luxembourg (5800 ECUs), and the lowest in Greece (1500 ECUs). Per capita expenditure in Italy, Belgium, Denmark, France and Germany is between 4000 ECUs and 5000 ECUs.

Figure 11.2 shows two distinct clusters. The first group consists of Greece, Portugal, Ireland and Spain. The second includes the Netherlands, Denmark, France, Belgium, Luxembourg, Italy and the UK. The differences between the two clusters should not, however, be exaggerated. Seen in an wider international context, and including, for example, Japan and the United States, there is more in common than separating these countries. The European Commission's Report

F.11.2

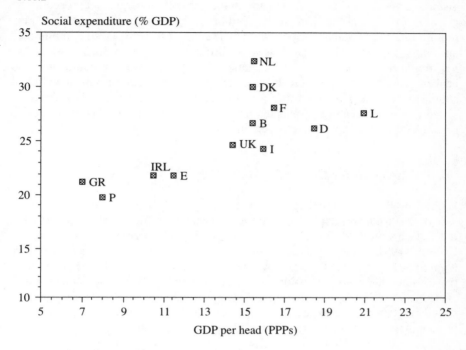

Figure 11.2: CEC (1994d), p. 42

on Social Protection clearly concludes that there are convergent trends in social protection expenditure within the Union. 'The coefficient of variation in the ratio of social expenditure to GDP, which measures divergence from the average, was 0.25 in 1980, but only 0.15 in 1991, indicating a significant convergence in levels' (CEC, 1994d, p. 43).

Outputs

Indicators of input (expenditure) provide a partial picture of convergent trends. It is equally important to consider the principles upon which allocative mechanisms are founded within member states and the policy outputs they achieve. The existence and salience of convergence between countries and through time cannot be mapped without indicators of outputs and (ultimately) outcomes. In this context, will the peripheral countries of the Union ever catch up with the northern core? Will the convergence of social protection systems follow the development of the Single Market? The answers depend on the role that social protection plays in developed economies and complex societies. As discussed above, it is a central tension in theories of convergence that economic growth can create not only prosperity, but hardship and exclusion, and these may require intervention and compensation. The support that displaced communities and individuals may need is made more difficult in complex societies because traditional relationships, family obligation and reciprocities are challenged and broken down. In such circumstances, and presuming a commitment to social solidarity and cohesion, there is a functional requirement for organized forms of social protection. The principles upon which they may be based and the precise organizational and delivery arrangements will vary greatly.

Prospects for Convergence

Within the European context a distinction may be drawn between Bismarckian and Beveridgean principles: the former, based on employment status, and the latter on a modified, but more inclusive, notion of citizenship. Chassard and Quintin (1992) have argued that these models are not as divergent as many would believe and that they are, over time, converging. They draw attention, on the one hand, to the expansion of social insurance schemes to include those previously excluded – including non-wage earners – and to trends towards supplementation of more generalized schemes through the involvement of the private market and occupationally based supplementation.

The European Union has narrow powers and competencies in the field of social policy, and even narrower competencies in the field of social protection (social security and health). Throughout its history, the Community has relegated social protection to the margins – but social protection could never be ignored. In the negotiations that led to the Treaty of Rome there was a debate, the echoes of which continue to resonate, between those (principally the French) who saw social protection as a form of indirect labour costs with a potential for distorting fair competition; and those (principally the Germans) who regarded indirect labour costs as only part of a wider picture that necessarily included fiscal policies, geographical location, industrial relations, social and cultural infra-structure. The argument revolves around the risks of what is now known as social dumping and the consequent need for the harmonization of social protection policies. There are two aspects to social dumping. The first relates to those circumstances in which companies facing higher employer costs (both direct and indirect) will be at a disadvantage compared to competitors in other countries facing lower costs. In such a scenario, it may be hypothesized that mobile capital will locate in countries or regions with low levels of social protection. The corollary is that in the interest of remaining competitive, there will be pressure to reduce levels of social protection in the more developed welfare states. A second variant of social dumping is better styled 'benefit tourism' where it is hypothesized that social security claimants will relocate to countries or regions with the highest levels of social protection. Despite fearful predictions to the contrary, there is little evidence that social dumping presents a serious threat to either the fair or ordered functioning of the market (Adnett, 1995).

Single European Market and the Wider Agenda

The Single European Act and its implementation as part of the 1992 project has given a stimulus to this debate. The optimism of the Cecchini Report (1988), which considered the medium and longer term implications of removing the remaining barriers to trade within the Union, suggested that there would be a significant boost in employment, economic output and a positive impact for social protection. Revenues would increase, unemployment and related deprivation would decline. But Cecchini (1988) exaggerated the benefits and underestimated the costs – the spillovers of economic integration – as was evidenced in the subsequent report by Padoa-Schioppa (1987). It was against this background that there was a renewed commitment to social policy in Europe: it was seen as being either a necessary facilitator of economic change and growth; or it was to be seen as an essential part of the strategy to meet the costs and to compensate for market completion.

Subsidiarity

The principle of subsidiarity, long regarded as a by-water of Catholic social doctrine, has been injected with a new lease of life (Spicker, 1991). A central aspect of the Maastricht Treaty and the EU White Paper on Social Policy, the principle requires that no decision should be taken at a higher level of political authority than is necessary for effective public policy; when applied in the sphere of social policy, this implies the reaffirmation of member state governments, and not the Council of Ministers, as the forum for decision making.

Although the principle of subsidiarity has further circumscribed the competence of the Union in respect of social policy, it is fully recognized that social protection measures impact on the functioning of the Single Market. A key function of social security policies is to ensure solidarity between those in the labour market and those who are not; against a background of technological change, it is the view of the Commission that social protection ensures not only social stability, but actually contributes to competitiveness. This is an area of high debate, and the evidence is inconclusive. A review by Pfaller *et al.* (1991) has looked at indicators of social expenditure and competitiveness, and has tentatively concluded that there is '... some evidence that states with higher levels of welfare statism (those with relatively high levels of social spending and which have remained closer to full employment than others) may have been less competitive in the late 1970s and early 1980s ...' (reported in Cochrane and Clarke, 1993, p. 247).

The Maastricht Treaty clearly declares in favour of a positive and pro-active role for social protection:

> The Community shall have as its task, by establishing a common market and an economic and monetary union and by implementing the common policies or activities referred to in Articles 3 and 3a, to promote throughout the Community a harmonious and balanced development of economic activities, sustainable and non-inflationary growth respecting of the environment, the high degree of convergence of economic performance, a high degree of employment and of social protection, the raising of the standard of living and quality of life, and economic and social cohesion and solidarity among Member States
>
> (quoted in CEC, (1994d), p. 11).

Two subsequent measures gave expression to this goal; the promise, however, has remained greater than the reality. The first measure was a Council Recommendation (92/442/EEC) on the convergence of social protection objectives and policies, which seeks to promote the convergence of policies around common objectives, while recognizing 'the integrity, independence and diversity of national systems'. The second measure was a Council Recommendation (92/441/EEC) on common criteria concerning sufficient resources and assistance in social protection systems. In both instances, key principles are elaborated, and the right to economic and social integration is asserted.

The Commission has set out the ways in which these Recommendations may be taken forward. First, it is necessary for all countries to take greater cognizance of structural change: in particular, to respond to demographic developments, especially the ageing population, with its implications for dependency ratios, pension systems and long term care needs. Additionally, they are to recognize that there is both instability and a need for flexibility in the labour market, with implications for work careers, social insurance cover and consequent entitlement to social protection. Some of these challenges are both a cause of, and a response to, high levels of unemployment. Other contextual issues include the emergence of new forms of poverty and social exclusion, new and changing family forms, and the continuing pursuit of equality between men and women in respect of social security entitlements.

Greater commitment to efficiency in the administration of social security systems, without compromising the rights or entitlements of claimants is something which all countries in the Union are considering: options include the removal of barriers to employment presently found in social protection systems in order to retain the support of those who contribute to funding social protection as well as those who receive support. There is a need to integrate social protection arrangements with other policies to reduce insecurity, and greater emphasis will be placed on preventing people having to have recourse to social security.

It is evident that the content and tone of recent policy documents coming from the Commission, including the White Papers, contain a 'new realism' and embody some of the rhetoric, as well as policies, of the United Kingdom Government. Far from being isolated and ignored within Europe, there are signs that the UK is having an influence and impact on thinking, especially in the field of social policy. But the full potential is not realized because the provisions of the Social Policy Agreement are increasingly invoked, and the UK is excluded from detailed policy formulation. This enables the Union to move forward, but at the same time denies the UK an opportunity to engage and debate with partners. Far from protecting British interests, such a position is a pretext for weakness; there is an abrogation of responsibility to shape Britain's future within the Union.

Structures and Visions for the Future

Britain's place within the European Union and the future direction of structures and policies are at the heart of debates within the Government, and will be the subject of the special Inter-Governmental Conference in 1996. There are common and emerging themes and trends in European social and political economy which make it exceedingly difficult for Britain (or any other country) to stand apart from the European venture. The integration of economies, the pursuit of convergent criteria – such as growth rates, unemployment levels, exchange rate stability – and the prospects for further enlargement involving the countries currently in transition, represent a continental and strategic future, which can be neither ignored nor reversed. The precise shape and scope of the developing European institutions and the extent of their responsibilities *vis-à-vis* nation states are uncertain, especially in the field of social policy. However, it is relatively easy to identify the possibilities, and several commentators have engaged in this speculation (Pieters, 1991; Chassard and Quintin 1992; Kleinman and Piachaud, 1993; Liebfried, 1994). Placed on a continuum, they range from minimalist to maximalist and the following have been set out by Kleinman and Piachaud (1993).

First, the clock could be turned back, and the Union could transform itself into a Free Trade customs union with no social policy; this is an unrealistic 'flat-earth' policy that would have been rejected by Adam Smith himself. But this vision does have its supporters. Second, there are those in favour of the so-called completion of the Single Market, and its further expansion to include central and eastern Europe. This widening of the European project would have inevitable consequences for its capacity to extend influence in the field of social policy. A third vision foresees a Federal Europe, of which there are two variants. On the one hand, a Federal Europe with a strong centre composed of a vigorous Commission and stream-lined European Council, or a weaker association of nation states in which regions and other policy actors would play an active part. Of central importance would be the principle and practice of subsidiarity, which would ensure a judicious balance of interests between centre and periphery. Finally, there are those, even yet, who have visions of a European Super State, developing a common European citizenship, committed to the prescription of firm and high social standards. For some, the occupational welfare arrangements provided for employees of the European Union provide an embryo of what might become a single welfare state. The possibilities are likely to be prosaic.

Social policy is an integral, if uncertain part, of the process of European integration; if the goal of a strong European market is wanted, then the social dimension must be acknowledged and accepted by Euro-sceptics and enthusiasts alike. The United Kingdom has the potential to help the future direction, and the 1996 Inter-Governmental Conference provides the setting. However, the British stance on many social policy questions, consistent with the opt-out from the European Charter and Social Chapter, risks the marginalization of British opinion and experience. There are trends toward the convergence of European economies and social structures but this does not require the development of common or harmonized social policies. The convergence of policy objectives and the commitment to achieve common and enhanced outcomes are not incompatible with a strong national identity – the current detachment of the British Government from European debates and decision making is an indication of weakness and not strength.

Note

1   The author would like to thank Neil Lunt and Anne Corden for comments on a draft of this chapter. Responsibility for the final version rests with the author alone.

References

ADNETT, N. (1995) 'Social dumping and European economic integration', *Journal of European Social Policy*, **5**(1), pp. 1–12.

CECCHINI, P. (1988) *The European Challenge 1992. The Benefits of a Single Market*, Aldershot: Wildwood House Ltd.

CEC (COMMISSION OF THE EUROPEAN COMMUNITIES) (1993) *Growth, Competitiveness, Employment. The Challenges and Ways Forward into the 21st Century*, White Paper, Luxembourg: European Commission.

CEC (COMMISSION OF THE EUROPEAN COMMUNITIES) (1994a) *European Social Policy A Way Forward for the Union*, White Paper COM (94) 333, Luxembourg: European Commission.

CEC (COMMISSION OF THE EUROPEAN COMMUNITIES) (1994b) *Employment in Europe*, Brussels: Commission of the European Communities.

CEC (COMMISSION OF THE EUROPEAN COMMUNITIES) (1994c) *The Demographic Situation in the European Union*, Brussels: Commission of the European Communities.

CEC (COMMISSION OF THE EUROPEAN COMMUNITIES) (1994d) *Social Protection in Europe 1993*, Brussels: Commission of the European Communities.

CEC (COMMISSION OF THE EUROPEAN COMMUNITIES) (1995) *Medium Term Social Action Programme*, Luxembourg: European Commission.

CHASSARD, Y. and QUINTIN, O. (1992) 'Social protection in the European Community: Towards a convergence of policies', *International Social Security Review*, **1–2**, pp. 91–108.

COCHRANE, A. and CLARKE, J. (Eds) (1993) *Comparing Welfare States*, London: Sage Publications.

ILO (INTERNATIONAL LABOUR OFFICE) (1995) *World Labour Report*, Geneva: ILO.

INGLEHART, R. (1990) *Culture Shift in Advanced Industrial Society*, Princeton, NJ: Oxford and Princeton University Press.

INGLEHART, R. and RABIER, J.R. (1986) 'Aspirations adapt to situation – but why are the Belgians so much happier than the French? A cross-cultural analysis of the subjective Quality of Life', in ANDERSON, F.M. (Ed.) *Research on the Quality of Life*, MI: University of Michigan Institute for Social Research.

KLEINMAN, M. and PIACHAUD, D. (1993) 'European social policy: some conceptions and choice', *Journal of European Social Policy*, **3**(1), pp. 1–19.

LIEBFRIED, S. (1994) 'The social dimension of the European Union: en route to positively joint sovereignty', *Journal of European Social Policy*, **4**(4), pp. 239–62.

PADOA-SCHIOPPA, T. (1987) *Efficiency, Stability and Equity*, Oxford: Oxford University Press.

PFALLER, A., GOUGH, I. and THERBORN, G. (Eds) (1991) *Can the Welfare State Compete? A Comparative Study of Five Advanced Capitalist Countries*, London: Macmillan.

PIETERS, D. (1991) 'Will "1991" lead to the coordination and harmonisation of social security?', in PIETERS, D. (Ed.) *Social Security in Europe*, Antwerp: Maklin.

SCANLON, T. (1993) 'Value, desire and quality of life', in NUSSBAUM, M.C. and SEN, A.K. (Eds) *The Quality of Life*, Oxford: Oxford University Press.

SPICKER, P. (1991) 'The principle of subsidiarity and the social policy of the European Community', *Journal of European Social Policy*, **1**(1), pp. 3–14.

Chapter 12

The Critical Welfare Agenda

Neil Small

Introduction

The contributors to this book illustrate well the diverse intellectual backgrounds brought to bear on welfare and policy issues. We can see links with social administration, political science and management studies, as well as with sociology and economics. Indeed many papers, as indeed much of the research literature in welfare and policy, demonstrate a hybrid quality in their intellectual antecedents. We also see a diversity of approach to the methodology of policy analysis – the qualitative and quantitative of course – but also differences in the starting point the writer takes, the deductive and the interpretive traditions are evident here. Contributors also show how valid it can be to locate agendas and issues in the broad context of whole systems, or to focus on the specifics of policy in one area.

The resulting combination of approaches does not lend itself to an easy synthesis. The evidence of such diversity does, though, prompt the question as to where research in welfare might develop. In this chapter, I will examine the changing structural and intellectual context of social research. Is this markedly different from that evident in the past? The question is raised as to how a reconciliation can be achieved between a push towards the esoteric, the reflexive and the uncertain in intellectual debate and a shift towards the instrumental in the social world of the researcher and research funder. Further, *can* the coalitions that characterize social research hold, indeed *should* they hold? Perhaps a break-up, and the challenges this would present, should be welcomed.

The Development of Social Research

If one consults the literature on the development of social research in the UK there is a strong emphasis on continuity in the character of research despite vastly different organizational structures.

> There is a strong historical continuity between the classic surveys of
> Booth, Rowntree ... and modern research ... including that of Abel-
> Smith and Townsend (Bulmer, 1982, p. 27).

Finch (1986) argues that the history of social research over 150 years has run
parallel to, and been closely intertwined with, the development of social policies
by central Government. But only one kind of social research has dominated;
'positivist in conception, quantitative in orientation, and often relying on the
social survey' (ibid., p. 1).

This has happened because of a belief by policymakers in the importance of
the 'unproblematic notion of objective facts', and the model of the researcher as
a technician who produces such facts but plays no part in decisions about
interpretation and use. Qualitative research has, at best, played a minor role,
perhaps because it has proved hard to convince that it meets the narrow criteria
for acceptability identified above (Finch, 1986, p. 223).

In the mid-1980s it was also possible to identify within universities a
situation in which applied social research had a lower status than 'pure'
disciplinary enquiry. There was less receptivity to highly organized, large scale
social research, and less ability to respond quickly to demands for rapid research.
Indeed, more social research was being carried out outside the universities than
in them (Bulmer *et al.*, 1986, p. xvii). However, there was some optimism about
the future. Bulmer *et al.* (1986) saw applied social research in the mid-1980s as
strong and healthy when compared to 1935 or 1960. The scale and variety of
activities was greater, the range of methodologies richer, the place of such
activities within Government was firmer, and the influence of social science on
the general culture was far reaching (Bulmer *et al.*, 1986, p. xix). Finch (1986)
saw the mid-1980s as evidencing a change in the mood of sociology towards less
overt hostility to empiricism and to policy oriented research, and a change in
social administration which saw it less wedded to a Fabian model and more
inclined to critical questioning.

Both Bulmer and Finch were demonstrating, in the main, supply side led
change. There was a cloud on the sunny horizon (a demand side cloud), although
not a very large cloud in Bulmer's 1987 estimation:

> It is possible to exaggerate the changes which have been made in recent
> years, to misinterpret somewhat the malevolence of the Reagan and
> Thatcher governments towards social science, and neglect the fact that
> applied social science is a fairly strongly entrenched, if small, sector of
> knowledge production in contemporary industrial societies. (Bulmer,
> 1987, p. xi)

What was the nature of that malevolence that Bulmer might not have been so
sanguine about had he known that the Thatcher and then Major regimes would

still be in place in the mid-1990s? In 1975 Margaret Thatcher argued that;

> a vital new debate is beginning, or perhaps an old debate is being renewed, about the proper role of government, the welfare state and the attitudes on which it rests ... (the debate centred on) the progressive consensus ... the doctrine that the State should be active on many fronts in promoting equality, in the provision of social welfare and in the redistribution of wealth and incomes. (quoted in Wicks, 1987, p. 22–3)

The leader of the Conservatives, then the Opposition party, made it clear that Margaret Thatcher was not part of this so called 'consensus'. Indeed, she is reported as saying, 'The other side have got an ideology ... we must have one as well' (Young, 1989, p. 406). We subsequently see unfolding an historic appropriation of the mantle of ideology from the left to the right with, at its height in the late 1980s, an ideologically invigorated right and impoverished left.

As the Thatcherite intention changed to action, following the 1979 Tory election victory, legislative and policy changes impacted on area after area of state activity. The cumulative result, by the mid-1980s, constituted a major change – even if its overall nature was subject to contested critiques. What became clear to all was that, in addition to the changes being profound, the impetus for change was not exhausted. The process continued in organizations already changed once, twice, or more as well as new areas succumbing to the juggernaut of this profoundly paradoxical conservatism.

Politics and Ideas

What has emerged is a welfare market place of sorts (see Le Grand, 1990). What role does social research have within it? John Maynard Keynes believed that the power of vested interests was vastly exaggerated compared with the gradual encroachment of ideas. Radika Desai (1994) has argued that in the 1970s and 1980s small bands of, seemingly marginal, neo-liberal and neo-conservative researchers turned their intuitions and prejudices into programmes and policies ready for adoption by politicians of the right throughout the world. In such a situation ideas, and the groups that propound them, in themselves take on the role of vested interests. It can consequently be argued that in the UK, and in many other countries, it is the vested interests of new right ideologues that define the parameters within which debates about the future of the welfare state take place.

These readings of the role of ideas in policymaking, are treated by some with scepticism. Neo-liberal and neo-conservative ideas did not gain influence because they were, in themselves, persuasive. Rather they were persuasive in so far as they were in accord with a trajectory of change within capitalism. This change included a restructuring of production – postfordism, a globalization of enterprise and markets – and a struggle between finance and manufacturing that the former was winning.

A second prompt to the sceptics comes from the paucity of the left to respond in any sustained way. Most people did not even wait for the third cock-crow before they disavowed a Marxism they had held tenaciously for many years. As for the parliamentary left, they appeared to decide that nothing should suggest that they held radical ideas, even though the country was being transformed by other sets of radical ideas. Recent debates following the publication of the Report of the Commission on Social Justice (1994) or the enthusiasm for Amitai Etzioni's communitarian agenda do little to reassure (Etzioni, 1993).

Returning to Thatcherism, Deakin (1987) has said that the totality of changes did not have a strong central focus; he cites the absence of links between changes in the benefits system and the tax system. But it has been argued by others, Anthony Gamble (1988) and Stuart Hall (1985) for example, that there is something at a more fundamental level that underpinned the changes. Gamble talks of the hegemonic project of Thatcherism, while Hall (1985) describes an 'authoritarian popularism' explaining:

> I hoped by adopting this deliberately contradictory term precisely to encapsulate the contradictory features of an emerging conjuncture: a movement towards a dominative and 'authoritarian' form of democratic class politics – paradoxically, apparently rooted in the transformism (Gramsci's term) of popularist discontents. (ibid., p. 118)

Within authoritarian popularism there may be a role for ideas that fuel the discontent upon which its ascendency depends. But once it has achieved some position of power it becomes hostile to criticism, and seeks to foreclose debate. Desai (1994) argues that Thatcherism, whatever its baneful effects did – at least – represent an attempt to link politics to ideas. Major has no such ambition, 'pragmatically cloaking in hypocritical moralism a continuing attack on public agency'.

The End of History?

There have also been arguments that the market ideology has triumphed, and in so doing has brought about 'the end of history' (Fukuyama, 1992). In such a situation, the idea of more programmes, from right or left, and hence a role for the intellectual organized in any sort of group must be questioned. Both the neo-liberal right and the Marxist left have 'end of history scenarios'. The dialectic ends, Hegel – even turned on his head – has his day!

Fukuyama (1992) develops the theme that there are two powerful forces at work in human history. These are 'the logic of modern science' and 'the struggle for recognition'. They will, over time, come together in such a way as to lead to a collapse of 'tyrannies'. Societies will be driven towards establishing liberal capitalist democracies, which he sees as the end state of the historical process.

From the left, the classical position is argued by Engels (1968). With the seizure of the means of production by society, 'The extraneous objective forces that have hitherto governed history pass under the control of man himself' (ibid., p. 68). The accumulation of knowledge would facilitate the more effective control of social forces in the interests of the people. Knowledge and power exist in close proximity in this future state. This end-point construct has been used as an intellectual and a practical justification for left academics in their engagement with social research.

It was only a small step from the Marxist left to the Fabian tradition that was dominant in the development of the academic discipline of social administration, and through it social policy. Fabianism was structured around empiricism and pragmatism. It also included a measure of idealism that change could be brought about by a combination of the production of evidence and the engagement of all concerned in rational debate. It is a tradition that is largely absent today. When we look at contemporary applied social research, the rationale is a defensive and not an innovative or programmatic one, I will return to this below.

There has not just been a case made for the end of history but also the end of universality. Postmodernism advocates pluralism in a world that is to be grasped as contingent, contextual and provisional. Human thought as a dialectical process in which a positive result can be achieved by hunting down and eliminating internal contradictions is rejected. Given such a scenario, what role is there for policy-related social science where the postmodern conversation is preferable to the analysis, the programme and the critique of modernist discourse (see Vincent, 1992, p. 4)?

Some social science has been profoundly touched by debates amongst structuralists and by deconstruction. Derrida (1994) is sceptical of the Fukuyama position not because he wants to argue that the idea of the end of history is inaccurate but that:

> [those] talking of the end of history now – after deconstruction – are like latecomers, a little as if it were possible still to take the last train after the last train and still be late for the end of history (ibid., p. 34).

If we have an end of history, at least as something amenable to systematic investigation and programmatic intervention, and an end of universalism as a meaningful construct, what then? We have to engage with social need. Even if we deconstruct it into an artefact of either history or modernity we have to address Derrida's (1994) challenge:

> Instead of singing the advent of the ideal of liberal democracy and the capitalist market in the euphoria of the end of history, instead of

celebrating the 'end of ideologies' and the end of the great emancipatory discourses, let us never again neglect this obvious macroscopic fact, made up of innumerable singular sites of suffering: no degree of progress allows one to ignore that never before, in absolute figures, never have so many men, women and children been subjugated, starved or exterminated on the earth. (ibid., p. 53)

Everything has not changed, and the need for both emancipatory theory and practice remains. The agenda becomes how to construct them without the foundations, or all the building blocks, we have looked to in the past. Postmodernism and deconstruction do not abrogate the need to engage with social need, nor do they deny the importance of change. In the same way as philosophies of praxis, or critical theory, they emphasize engagement and change rather than programmes and 'solutions'.

We see in this brief review of the political context that impinges on social research two key questions that we must return to:

1   If political pragmatism has followed hegemonic change does this foreclose intellectual debate, at least in so far as it might impact on policymaking?
2   The triumph of one ideology, or the break in the dominance of single ideas or meta-narratives might end history, as it has been constructed in modernity, but it does not end need. How can we generate the methodological imagination to address this new world?

The Organization of Social Research

There is a danger when bemoaning the current state of social research to set up a golden age myth. Wherever we sit we can usually look back and say things were better before (see Pearson, 1983, pp. 7–11).

We may see the past as better for *us*, rather than for social research *per se*. This can involve a discussion about quantity and quality in terms of social research. There are more people than ever in university education, research centres are full to overflowing with staff, new journals spring up, attendance at conferences (and papers submitted) keeps rising.

The argument posed in opposition to this apparent healthy state is that an atmosphere of unease and insecurity surrounds social research. Insecurity in the position of staff, terms and conditions of employment; control over the subjects of research; over the approach and method allowed; and over the ownership and dissemination of findings. The NHS Research and Development programme is illustrative. This programme is funding more research even though there is a shortage of skilled researchers and continuing blocks between the generation of research findings and recommendations, and the ability and the willingness of purchasers and providers of health care to implement them (Maynard, 1994).

Has the capacity of social research to exercise policy influence declined? A persuasive case can be made for the long term failure of health policy research to influence policy. David Hunter (1988), talking about the years 1974 to 1988, has argued that 'social science research has failed to inform any of the changes in the NHS over the past 14 years'. Assumptions made about the efficacy of particular proposals and solutions have been grounded in little or no research, and have sought instead to establish their creditability with reference to somewhat outmoded theories of organization and management (Hunter, 1988, p. 538).

Pollitt *et al.* (1990) have argued that as Government policies are not research led, they are not keen on research uncovering uncertainties and ambiguities. Even where there is research, it may not be done when most needed, and may be concerned only with what is immediately relevant and useful. Walker (1989) sees the nature of commissioned social policy research as being much altered. There is less concern with discovering new problems, or in documenting them. Now the concern is with the implementation of policy, and how such policies can be more cost effective.

Although it has never been easy to conduct research into currently sensitive policy areas, there is now accumulating evidence that various forms of resistance to scholarly investigation are on the increase (Webb, 1992). The detailed form of resistance can be listed: ignoring inconvenient studies; manipulating statistics; refusing publication; effectively embargoing funding for individual researchers; attacking the motives of individual researchers (Pollitt *et al.*, 1990, p. 169).

It is, of course, not just these more overt forms of resistance but the general atmosphere in which researchers, and would-be researchers, contemplate the parameters of the possible that conditions what is attempted.

The Context of Research in Universities

Within higher education we have researchers working individually or in research centres with, in the main, short term contracts. Much of the work so generated is best categorized as audit, not research. In essence, the difference is that the former is concerned to examine how effectively an intervention has been applied, whereas the latter is concerned to identify or confirm new facts relating to specific problems (Smith, 1992; Bull, 1993).

But perhaps critical research can go on outside funded research, in the ongoing life of established academics. There is a myth in research centres, that academics in teaching departments can indulge themselves in obscure theoretical debate; and a myth in teaching departments that research centres explore the frontiers of advanced methodology. In reality, while researchers are beset by the control exercised by funders, those academics in teaching departments are just about surviving increased student numbers, the realization that the extra hardship impoverished and/or indebted students face increases the support they need, the growth in administrative burdens, and the pressure of research selectivity exercises.

From the viewpoint of those wishing to develop applied, and inter-disciplinary, research, Research Selectivity Exercises have an invidious impact on the nature of academic activity. Let us consider economics as an example. The academic output of economics departments is assessed as to its merit according to the journals material is published in (there are other considerations as well but this one is the bottom line). This prompts a disproportionate interest in writing clever pieces, whose erudition and originality can only be appreciated by other economists. Industrial economists, for example, no longer aspire to write about firms or business, rather they write about economic game theory. Economists are speaking only to themselves in an increasingly rarefied and esoteric language.[1]

Reporting on Research

The history of applied social research and its relationship with the Government and with the academic community has been shaped by a number of key reports. The Clapham Report (1946) identified a role for the Government in sponsoring the development of social science. Earmarked grants to universities followed, although they were more facilitative of an expansion of teaching rather than research. The Heyworth Report (1965) looked at sponsorship of social research by the Government and the establishment of the Social Science Research Council followed (its name was changed to the Economic and Social Research Council in 1983). The Rothschild Report (1982) underlined the necessary coexistence of both fundamental and applied research.

Research into social care, social work and the health service have been subject to scrutiny in a number of reports in recent years. I will comment in some detail on three of these. A consideration of these reports reveals a new emphasis on the dissemination of research findings and the emergence of the primacy of the 'customer'. But the approach gleaned from reading all the reports is not entirely consistent.

In 1991 the Department of Health decided to create 14 regional bureauc-racies to manage NHS research and development, alongside a centrally commissioned programme (Department of Health, 1991). The reforms to the then existing programme were ostensibly designed to bring research and service delivery closer together; to emphasize 'what works' in health care, to generate information it was felt would be of central concern to both purchasers and providers. The Department hoped that research would involve the contribution of a wide range of disciplines and subjects. But early experience saw the dominance of medicine; all Regional Directors of Research were clinicians and, for example, the first Regional Research and Development Committee set up in the north west region had representatives of many medical specialities but no social scientist. The danger was that social science would be seen as optional technical support to clinical health research.

The second impact of the 1991 reform was to set in motion the end of core funding to the 13 Department of Health research units then in existence. The Williams Report (1992) argued that the number and spread of the existing units was too wide, and the disciplinary composition too narrow, to meet the requirements of the new research and development strategy. The intention was to divert funds to three or four new grand centres. These would be multi-disciplinary, an approach the Williams committee and others (Clarke and Kurinczuk, 1992) saw as the best way to carry out health and personal social services research.

An alternative approach, suggested by Maynard and Sheldon (1992), would be to recognize that neither health service research nor medicine are, in themselves, disciplines. They are subjects. Perhaps units with a 'lead' discipline and a strong disciplinary base may have greater intellectual coherence and anchorage to carry out quality work. Collaboration would not be within units as much as between units. This is an argument for diversity rather than multi-disciplinarity.

The Williams Report (1992) was predicated on the belief that the current organization of research was not serving the NHS as well as it might. There was a lack of focus and strategy, and a poor record in the dissemination of results. But perhaps that was the fault of the NHS in general, and the Department of Health in particular, and not the research. The House of Lords Select Committee on Science and Technology (1988) identified a lack of coherent policy, or evident coordination, in Department of Health research. In general, in the 1980s, health policy was dominated by change and not by planning or strategy. Research reflected short term needs. Maynard and Sheldon (1992) have suggested that a diversity of the research base may have, in effect, protected the research community from policy oscillations.

The current wish to concentrate on fewer centres may not serve the Department well, because the units may be less responsive. They may not service research well in that they will be even more vulnerable to pressure from the Department (sums allocated will be too large to come from any alternative source). They may not serve researchers well because they may feel cut off from their disciplinary roots. Greater size, in this scenario, produces – perhaps paradoxically – more uniformity and vulnerability.

Smith (1994) claimed that personal social services research has had a significant impact on policy, for example, in informing both the 1989 Children's Act and the guidance on its implementation. However other areas, community care research for example, has had more resources allocated to it but without the same impact on policy. It may be that this is, as Smith (1994) suggests, because community care is essentially enacted across the interface of health and social care, and personal social services research has not well addressed that interface.

Indeed, as we look further it appears that the influence of research on the Children's Act, which is so often cited, is an exception and not the rule. Much of the literature on the impact of research looks to the difficulties inherent in this activity as it pertains to the personal social services. Much research is diffuse, being built up from varied evidence, with outcomes presented as something to do with a balance struck between gains and losses (see Pahl, 1992). There is an undeveloped academic framework, and not sufficiently developed links between academia, managers and practitioners.

Smith (1994) also recognized that the conceptual framework of the social services, and hence of personal social services research, is relatively undeveloped. The remedy his report offer, looks to more enhanced dissemination, closer cooperation between field and academia, and a development of research literacy in professional and managerial training. What it does not address is the vacuum at the heart of their analysis. While it is possible to enhance all the areas they identify, the impression is that what you will be enhancing is a chimera. What Smith (1994) is offering is cosmetic. It is both the tentativeness of the alliance of disciplines that make up personal social services research, and the absence of theoretical development that must be addressed.

The final report I will comment on was published in September 1994. Chaired by Professor Anthony Culyer (Culyer, 1994), it looked at new ways of supporting research and development in the NHS. The report argues that it is essential to separate funds for research and development from funds for other activities. Culyer (1994) is proposing prioritizing a national research strategy, led by the NHS but encompassing other research funders. There must be a research function over and above that defined as being in the interests of purchasers and providers seeking to improve value for money, and enhance managerial efficiency and accountability. The implications of this report are twofold. First that the implementation of 'Working for Patients', without the adjustments he is calling for, is not in the interests of medium and long term research agendas within the health service. Second, that there has to be a centralized research sponsor. In the era of the market this appears as a dirigist interloper! Taken together, these reports show common concerns with effective dissemination. But there are a number of points of different emphasis:

1   On the relationship between purchasers, providers and research: there needs to be a concern with what works for purchasers and providers (1991 report): research cannot be just for purchasers and providers, there is a longer term agenda (Culyer, 1994).
2   Multidisciplinary research: there is a general agreement that the nature of the subject area requires multidisciplinary research. But it is not clear how best to pursue this – multidisciplinarity can be claimed even if there is an overwhelmingly dominant partner. It can also undermine the professional

self-confidence of some groups. For effective diversity, and the clear added value of bringing disciplines together, one needs participants confident in the integrity of their own discipline.

3   On who leads on research agendas: there is a difference between keeping research and service delivery close together and the Culyer point that a centralized research sponsor is needed to ensure the medium and long term agendas. It is doubtful that the Smith agenda of a more developed conceptual framework and better links between academics, managers and practitioners can be achieved if it is the managers and practitioners who lead.

4   On the balance between theoretical and applied research: the balance swings, first in 1991 towards purchaser and provider led initiatives – an emphasis on what works, through to the Culyer (1994) reservations about such an arrangement addressing the sorts of strategic questions that must be asked. A second level of tension, between the interpretive and analytic, is evident in the subtext of discussions about multidisciplinary services requiring multidisciplinary research teams. It is also inherent in Smith's (1992) concerns about undeveloped conceptual frameworks.

Theorizing Social Research

I have now looked at both the changing political context of social research and the institutional context within which much research is carried out. In this third substantive section about influences on social research I will examine the nature of theoretical debate in sociology and economics – both how these debates are shaping the discipline and how they contribute to collaboration in applied social research.

I have argued above that amidst changing times we get, in the main, a new approach – defensive social research. George and Miller (1994) warn that the affordable welfare state will gradually decline into the residual welfare state, as much by default through inadequate funding as through deliberate policy. Glennerster (1993, p. 22) has argued that the task of social policy is to design 'the most humane system of residual welfare we can'. The importance of recognizing the gap between policy and implementation feature in Hill's (1993) work. Page and Deakin (1993) survey the wreckage of universalism and identify the way that welfare regimes may be reshaped for survival at the end of the twentieth century.

Alongside defensive social policy there is an approach to the ascendency of the market philosophy that seeks to construct a new social policy, free of the state. Let's call this offensive social policy. Green, for example, argues for a revival of voluntary traditions of welfare provision. These are to be encouraged by operating a presumption against public sector provision. He argues that the 'dependent poor' should be given practical help, which he claims is an approach superior to 'mere alms giving' (Green, 1993, p. 147). Anderson has argued that an end to rationality, to principles and reasoned enquiry in decisions about state welfare policy, means that social policy is 'left without its field of application and the status which derived from it' (Anderson, D. 1990, p. 43).

Cahill (1994) argues that a new social policy is now needed which takes cognizance of the end of the classic welfare state, of the information revolution, of globalization and the end of the cold war. This new social policy should be constructed around a 'social life analysis'. By this he means an analysis of communicating, viewing, travelling, shopping, working and playing. It is, though, in his presentation a peculiarly untheorized 'new' social policy.

We have, in Cahill's (1994) work, a good example of an area where theoretical debate exists, it is just that it appears to have been misplaced in his book. Indeed, Cahill's (1994) presentation of social policy via an examination of everyday life is consistent with pluralist critiques of the redundancy of universality as a defining concept in the late twentieth century.

The danger in casting social policy adrift from theory is that it becomes vulnerable, intellectually as well as institutionally to short-termism and anti-intellectualism. The demands for policy oriented research risk setting up the sorts of relations between funders and researchers where funders, solely, decide what are appropriate research questions, and where specifications are so tight as to pre-empt any critical input. The end point for funders is that they get told what they pay to hear, and for researchers and research centres, that they judge 'success' as the generation of a production line of reports.

While social policy has been engaging with creating defensive configurations, economics saw a struggle between an academic establishment that was still occupied, in some of its higher echelons, by people sympathetic to Keynesianism and by the resurgence of the neo-classical tradition. Within the hegemonic project of Thatcherism economics occupied a significant place. It became something of a battle ground. The academic establishment used those things at its disposal, publicly creating distance between policy and theory – a letter signed by 364 economists against Mrs Thatcher's economic policies, or withholding approval and recognition – Oxford University refusing to award an honorary degree to Mrs Thatcher for example (Desai, 1994, p. 62). The Thatcherite response had three components;

1 underlining ascendency in policy and thereby implying the irrelevance of the critical academic. Keynesianism had been influential specifically because it dominated both policy and academic debate.
2 Changing the context of academic economics as a sub-agenda in the changing structure of higher education.
3 Pushing ahead faster in those areas of economics not as integrated into the higher education establishment, development economics as practised by the IMF and World Bank for example (Anderson, D. 1990).

The struggle, when carried out over some years, was not an even one. By 1992 we can recognize that, as Granovetter (1992) has argued, there had been a return to dominance by the pure neo-classical tradition, after a period of contention with competing paradigms. There had also been an attempt by economists to greatly broaden their subject matter. Some economists have adopted an increasingly triumphalist stance. Hirshleifer (1985) wrote about the expanding domain of economics arguing that 'economics really does constitute the universal grammar of social science' (ibid., p. 53).

Neither the triumph of neo-classicism nor the expansion of the claimed sphere of competence of economics encourages economists to share the shifting concerns of their interpretive colleagues. Those methods that adopt a particularly mathematical approach claim rigour and relevance. It is a claim that can appeal, but it is sustained only if we uncritically accept the specific set of assumptions the method operates within. Charles and Webb (1986, p. 69) describe how such approaches frequently assert, or assume, a generalizable preference ordering. They also presume some sort of macro-level equilibrium. It is an approach that takes a narrow view of human motivation, assuming the widespread existence of rational utility maximization, and only reluctantly acknowledging the existence of other cognitive procedures such as habit, loyalty, or allegiance to some collective or cooperative ideal.

There are some economists who exist outside the dominant neo-classical tradition (Lunt *et al.*, 1994). It can be argued that the contribution they make positions them closer to the 'traditional' social research alliance. Austrian economics, for example, re-emerged as one of the alternatives to Keynesianism in the 1970s (Kirzner, 1973). Von Hayek was one of the gurus claimed by the new right and his, and the Austrian School's, approach to the entrepreneurial spirit and to the dynamic market of alteration and change links with the agendas of social research. There are also critiques of the market, developed by an approach identified as the 'New Economic Sociology'. Here, there is a recognition that markets operate through networks of social actors and groups, and that the nature of this interaction supports and influences economic exchange (Granovetter and Swedberg, 1992).

The introduction of non-individualistic and non-'rational' factors, and the possibility of debating the ethics of economics, present two challenges to neo-classical and rational choice theory. Gordon Tullock, over many years, has developed the argument that in both economics and politics what drives people is self-interest as they seek to maximize their advantage (Tullock, 1965). This approach has been very influential on both sides of the Atlantic. In the US it is argued, albeit by Tullock (ibid.), that 90 per cent of economists are 'rational choice types, though the same cannot be said of political scientists. The bulk of political scientists remain devoted to old fashioned ideas' (quoted in *Times Higher Education Supplement*, 17 February 1995). Much sociological theory has, to a considerable degree, been fashioned in reaction to assumptions about human rationality. Occasional forays have been made in pursuing rational choice theory in sociology (see Abell, 1991), but such approaches remain largely marginal.

'Rational choice' is now under sustained attack. Green and Shapiro (1994) have criticized its use in politics, arguing that it offers an appeal to people seeking the signs and symbols of 'science', but in effect it substitutes an empty formalism for real advances. In economics there are a number of directions of criticism. In effect, and particularly in the UK, other factors are being added into market models – ignorance, inconsistency, altruism and the panoply of social – that is non-individualistic, influences on economic behaviour. As Walker (1995) has argued, these developments have 'taken the form of seeking to admit a limited dose of reality into market models'. Some economists are developing a variant of rational choice theory, called 'gaming', carried out via experimental work in which people are set questions and are faced with choices, and the extent to which they maximize utility, or behave consistently in their preferences, is recorded. An Economic and Social Research Council programme, led by Peter Taylor-Gooby of Kent University, is looking at cultural factors and group influences that feed economic behaviour.

Second, there is the increasingly cited work of Amitai Etzioni, an economist whose approach appears to have been enthusiastically embraced by the Blair Labour Party in the UK, especially by Shadow Chancellor Gordon Brown, and by elements of the Clinton administration in the US. Etzioni, in a series of books, has been seeking to foster a debate on the moral dimension of economics (Etzioni, 1988) and the communitarian agenda within which economics must be located (Etzioni, 1993). Etzioni is presenting the case for a new paradigm, embracing the communitarian and moral. It is a paradigm that he hopes will move the discipline of economics on from what he identifies as the present struggle between neo-classical approaches, which are applied not just to economics but to the full array of social relations from crime to the family, and the social-conservative approach which looks to strong authority to control dangerous impulses.

In considering the potential to perpetuate the alliance between analytic and interpretive discourses the Austrian school, New Economic Sociology, critical approaches to rational choice and Etzioni's putative paradigm all appear to offer possibilities. But, as yet, this would not be an alliance that encompassed either the core of the intellectual debate in economics, or that addressed the main route of influence for economics on policy. Neo-classical economics, in triumphalist mode, is not likely to prioritize an alliance with the interpretive social sciences. It can also be argued that it is not economics, as such, that has an impact on policy, but accountancy. Bottom line cost counting is not economics.[2]

The Impact of Postmodernism

There is the potential for a renewed debate on theory, arising out of attempts within social research to address the challenges of postmodernism. But the different components that go into making up the applied social research hybrid have engaged with postmodernism in very varying degrees. Taylor-Gooby (1994) points to the difference between the interpretive social sciences (see Schutz, 1967), including sociology, which have engaged with postmodernism, and the analytic, including economics, which have not. He is concerned that the impact of theory, in this case, may be to widen a divide between these two collaborating disciplines in social research.

Taylor-Gooby believes that 'social policy research is concerned to generate high quality objective knowledge that can be deployed in social planning' (Taylor-Gooby, 1994, p. 387). He argues that postmodernism offers a challenge to social policy in both theory and practice. Social policy has stressed universal themes of inequality and privilege and a practice ethos based on rational analysis oriented towards society-wide Government provision. Postmodernism, as I have argued above, has no place for the programmatic or the universal.

There are two ways of moving forward. First, argue that modernity is still with us. Or, second, accept that we live in postmodern times and develop social research accordingly. Taylor-Gooby is in good company in seeking the first route. He argues that there is still a place for the established concerns in a world where 'the trend towards economic liberalism is the nearest approximation to a universal theme in world affairs' (Taylor-Gooby, 1994, p. 388). Berman (1982) sees the essence of modernity as change, and sees change inherent in the immense capacities of technology and in the energy of the city. Giddens (1992) argues that prophecies of a transition to postmodernity are premature. We live in 'high modernity' he says. It is a place where the systemic weaknesses of a rationally based order are increasingly apparent. Yet the grip of industrial capitalism on everyday life is as vigorous as ever, and the capacity of national governments to control a technology of violence and to use increasingly sophisticated methods of social control is also evident. Doyal and Gough argue for universality from the standpoint of needs:

> We all have the same needs which are real and objective. Needs are therefore conceptualised independently of a particular social environment. (1991, p. 9, see also Hewitt, 1993)

Finally, Habermas places social movements within the framework of a universalist communicative ethic. As such, he retains the possibility of a universal emancipatory programme that transcends its specific, and apparently different, manifestations in a number of sites of praxis; feminism, ecology, the struggle in post-colonialist societies and so on (see for example, Dews, 1986).

Taylor-Gooby's argument about the universal theme of economic liberalism is open to empirical criticism. Indeed he rehearses some of the arguments:

> Just as the universalising themes of the grand narrative have frag-
> mented, so the universalising archetype of the manufacturing enterprise
> has been replaced by flexible specialisation and the idea that workers are
> marshalled, unified and standardised as a class by the demands of the
> assembly line replaced by the pluralist patterns of communities of
> interest. (Taylor-Gooby, 1994, pp. 397–8)

In many different areas of life we see the grand narratives of the natural and the
social sciences failing. This is evident in biology, in physics, in astronomy as
well as in business and commerce. In information technology the new
possibilities herald, for optimists like McLuhan: 'the end of Western analytic
reason (homogeneous, standard and linear) and the dawn of a new age, a return
to lost, pre-Gutenberg values' (Wollen, 1993, pp. 66–7).

In contrast, Baudrillard's pessimistic vision sees the new technology as: 'an
extension of analytic reason, through which digitalization becomes the final
culmination of a process of alienation' (Wollen, 1993, pp. 67).

In the social sciences, the days of a 'Weberian emphasis on confidence in the
rationality of state administration' have gone (Taylor-Gooby, 1994, p. 393). Yet
Taylor-Gooby still argues for economic liberalism as a universal theme. It might
be more convincingly constructed as a manifestation of the absence of defining
themes rather than a theme in itself, as evidence of the postmodernist case and
not as its contradiction.

Turning to the second possible response to postmodernism, that is considering those features that have a relevance for the development of a postmodern
approach to social research, we start with postmodernism's concern to 'cultivate
an awareness of the plurality and contingency of human interests' (Hewitt, 1993,
p. 55). It concerns itself with local determinism and small narratives (Lyotard,
1984), and recognizes that societies function reflexively with the 'increasing
ability to act on itself' (Touraine, 1981, p. 2). If one starts with such a point of
view, then imposing order on data, generalizing, constructing meanings, is
problematic. The panoply of qualitative analysis needs to illuminate people's
reflexive subjectivity, and not seek to impose a hierarchy of meaning. Ethnog-
raphy as an approach remains. It can be supported by quantitative data, but not
used the other way around.

An example will help illustrate. In the area of population health research and
practice one needs to move from seeking to construct models from surveys of
individual risk behaviour. Rather, one should consider social causation and
cultural influences, using qualitative research methods (see the 'Leeds Declaration' Nuffield Institute for Health, Leeds University; also Eskin, 1994). Professor
Jonathan Mann of Harvard has recently argued that research into HIV and AIDS

should also adopt such an agenda (Plenary address, AIDS Impact – Conference, Brighton, July 1994).

In relation more specifically to social welfare, Williams (1992) has suggested a number of different areas for study, including:

> The ways in which needs for universal welfare provision may be resolved with the need to meet diversity and difference, both at the level of policy planning and at the level of collective action around welfare demands and at the level of individual and collective empowerment to articulate needs. (Williams, F., 1992, p. 210)

The problem, evident in Williams's position but endemic in the defensive social policy discussed above, is of not going far enough. It is as if the attraction of universalism and of programmatic agendas exercises a remorseless pull.

Going all the way would see a reorientation towards knowledge and power. An example from the world of politics will help illustrate the difference. Burbach has described the postmodern rebellion in Chiapas, Mexico.

> A postmodern strategy aims not at seizing power but at changing the relationship of forces throughout Mexican society. The objective is to spark a broad based movement of civil society . . . that will transform the country from the bottom up. (1994, p. 113)

The Mexican peasant well knows that overthrowing one ruler without doing anything about the nature of rule leaves them, very soon, in the same position they were before.

Conclusion

I have argued in this paper that the recent past saw a brief period in which the power of ideas had an impact on the programmes of the right. This was followed by an evocation of the end of history, which served as a rationale for foreclosure of debate. Foreclosure was, in part, carried out via the manipulation of the means of academic production – via funding, contracts and conditions of work. But the end of history, profoundly Eurocentric as such an position is, ignores as Derrida (1994) has reminded us – and as any news bulletin confirms, the continuing need for an analysis of inequality and oppression.

I included a brief review of the changing formal structure of research in the UK university sector, and the way that this impacts upon both the sorts of questions that are asked, and who is available to ask them. I then turned to debates concerning theorizing social change. I have argued that to engage with postmodernism involves both opportunity and challenge. It is possible to develop an emancipatory agenda without slipping back into programmatic universalism.

At the beginning of this chapter I indicated that I would address two underlying questions. Can the coalition that has characterized social research so far hold? My conclusion is that the pressures are such that it cannot. There are some caveats because within economics, in particular, there are contributors whose approach sits close to the concerns of sociology and within the research community there is some recognition that a concern with the subjective meaning of social action benefits from a context that includes an analytic appreciation of social and economic structures. Further, as I have presented, there is a great deal of debate as to the nature of modernity. Is it continuing, 'late', or 'post'? The way we answer this will shape our response to the second question I posed at the outset, should the coalition hold?

I have considered above the challenge and opportunity of postmodernism. Postmodernism is intellectually centrifugal, and the social research coalition tends towards the centripetal. If postmodernism wins the day we can expect a series of contingent associations, not really alliances and certainly not affiliations. If we are convinced by the case that there is no centre, and so no need to hold a centre together, then we conclude that the alliance can be dispensed with, without real loss and without our tears.

One doubt remains however; what now is the role of the intellectual, or rather if we are mindful of Gramsci's distinction that all are intellectuals, but not all in society have the function of intellectuals, of those in society that carry on this function (Gramsci, 1971, pp. 8–9)? Anderson seems to argue that, in the social sciences at least, intellectuals are those who concern themselves with the study of social reality (Anderson, P. 1992, p. 50). Debray adds, as a necessary component of the intellectual, a social engagement (Debray, 1981, p. 32). Berger and Luckmann (1967) allow that an intellectual can be an expert, but what they call a true intellectual is not someone who adds expertise in a socially legitimizing way. Rather, it is someone whose expertise is not wanted by society.

I have argued above that the idea of social reality, and the reality of social engagement and the independent critical stance are problematic. The nature of intellectual debate, the circumstances of intellectual production and the context of social debate all compromise the opportunity to pursue such an intellectual agenda. Rather, at least in the academic disciplines of economics, sociology and in the hybrid of social research we see the danger of the disappearance of the intellectual, replaced by those concerned with the insular, esoteric, calling of the academic (see Jacoby, 1987) or by those pursuing agendas defined from above which makes applied social research akin to a service industry.

Neil Small

Notes

1 Thanks to Professor Keith Hartley for pointing this out to me.
2 Thanks to Roy Carr-Hill who reminded me of this distinction.

References

ABELL, P. (Ed.) (1991) *Rational Choice Theory*, London: Edward Elgar Publishing.
ANDERSON, D. (1990) 'The state of the social policy debate', in MANNING, N. and UNGERSON, C. (Eds) *Social Policy Review 1989–1990*, Harlow: Longmans. pp. 30–43.
ANDERSON, P. (1990) 'A culture in contraflow', *New Left Review*, **180**, **182**, pp. 41–78, pp. 85–137.
ANDERSON, P. (1992) *English Questions*, London: Verso.
BERGER, P.L. and LUCKMANN, T. (1967) *The Social Construction of Reality*, Harmondsworth: Penguin.
BERMAN, M. (1982) *All That is Solid Melts into Air*, London: Verso.
BULL, A. (1993) 'Audit and research', *British Medical Journal*, **306**, p. 67.
BULMER, M. (1982) *The Uses of Social Research*, London: George Allen and Unwin.
BULMER, M. (Ed.) (1987) *Social Science Research and Government*, Cambridge: Cambridge University Press.
BULMER, M., BUNTING, K.G., BLUME, S.S., CARLEY, M. and WEISS, C.H. (1986) *Social Science and Social Policy*, London: Allen and Unwin.
BURBACH. R. (1994) 'Roots of the postmodern rebellion in Chiapas', *New Left Review*, **205**, pp. 113–24.
CAHILL, M. (1994) *The New Social Policy*, Oxford: Blackwell.
CHARLES, S. and WEBB, A. (1986) *The Economic Approach to Social Policy*, Brighton: Wheatsheaf.
CLAPHAM REPORT, (1946) *Report of the Committee on the Provision for Social and Economic Research*, Cmnd 6868, London: HMSO.
CLARKE, M. and KURINCZUK, J.J. (1992) 'Health Services Research: a case of need or special pleading', *British Medical Journal*, **304**, pp. 1675–6.
CULYER, A. (1994) *Supporting Research and Development in the NHS*, London: HMSO.
DEAKIN, N. (1987) *The Politics of Welfare*, London: Methuen.
DEBRAY, R. (1981) *Teachers, Writers and Celebrities: The Intellectuals of Modern France*, London: Verso.
DEPARTMENT OF HEALTH (1991) *Research for Health – A Research and Development Strategy for the NHS*, London: Department of Health.
DERRIDA, J. (1994) 'Spectres of Marx', *New Left Review*, **205**, pp. 31–58.
DESAI, R. (1994) 'Second-hand dealers in ideas: think-tanks and Thatcherite hegemony', *New Left Review*, **203**, pp. 27–64.
DEWS, P. (1986) *Habermas: Autonomy and Solidarity. Interviews with Jurgen Habermas*, London: Verso.
DOYAL, L. and GOUGH, I. (1991) *A Theory of Human Need*, Basingstoke: Macmillan.
ENGELS, F. (1968) *Socialism: Utopian and Scientific*, Moscow: Progress Publishers.

ESKIN, F. (1994) 'The Leeds Declaration': refocusing public health research for action, *Critical Public Health*, **5**(3), pp. 39–44.

ETZIONI, A. (1988) *The Moral Dimension. Towards a New Economics*, New York: The Free Press.

ETZIONI, A. (1993) *The Spirit of Community: Rights, Responsibilities and the Communitarian Agenda*, New York: Crown Publishing Group.

FINCH, J. (1986) *Research and Policy*, London: Falmer Press.

FUKUYAMA, F. (1992) *The End of History and the Last Man*, Harmondsworth: Penguin.

GAMBLE, A. (1988) *The Free Economy and the Strong State*, London: Macmillan.

GEORGE, V. and MILLER, S. (Eds) (1994) *Social Policy Towards 2000: Squaring the Welfare Circle*, London: Routledge.

GIDDENS, A. (1992) *The Transformation of Intimacy*, Cambridge: Polity Press.

GLENNERSTER, H. (1993) Paying for welfare: issues for the nineties, in PAGE. R. and DEAKIN, N. (Eds) (1993) *The Costs of Welfare*, Aldershot: Avebury, pp. 13–28.

GRAMSCI, A. (1971) *Selections from the Prison Notebooks*, London: Lawrence and Wishart.

GRANOVETTER, M. (1992) 'Economic institutions as social constructions: a framework for analysis', *Acta Sociologica*, **35**, pp. 3–11.

GRANOVETTER, M. and SWEDBERG, R. (1992) *The Sociology of Economic Life*, Oxford: Westview Press.

GREEN, D.G. (1993) *Reinventing Civil Society: The Rediscovery of Welfare without Politics*, London: IEA.

GREEN, D.P. and SHAPIRO, I. (1994) *Pathologies of Rational Choice Theory: A Critique of Applications in Political Science*, New Haven, CT: Yale University Press.

HALL, S. (1985) 'Authoritarian Popularism', *New Left Review*, **151**, pp. 115–23.

HEWITT, M. (1993) 'Social movements and social need: problems with postmodern political theory', *Critical Social Policy*, **37**, pp. 52–74.

HEYWORTH REPORT (1965) *Report of the Committee on Social Studies*, Cmnd 2660, London: HMSO.

HILL, M. (1993) *Understanding Social Policy*, 4th Edn, Cambridge: Blackwell.

HIRSHLEIFER, J. (1985) 'The expanding domain of economics', *American Economic Review*, **85**, pp. 53–68.

HOUSE OF LORDS SELECT COMMITTEE ON SCIENCE AND TECHNOLOGY (1988) *Priorities in Medical Research*, **1**, London: HMSO.

HUNTER, D. (1988) 'The impact of research on restructuring the British National Health Service', *The Journal of Health Administration Education*, **6**(3), Summer pp. 537–53.

JACOBY, R. (1987) *The Last Intellectuals : American Culture in the Age of the Academe*, New York: Farrar Straus and Giroux Inc.

KIRZNER, I.M. (1973) *Competition and Entrepreneurship*, Chicago: University of Chicago Press.

LE GRAND, J. (1990) *Quasi-markets and Social Policy*, Studies in Decentralisation and Quasi-markets, **1**, School for Advanced Urban Studies: University of Bristol.

LUNT, N., MANNION, R. and SMITH, P. (1994) 'Theories of the market: the case of community care', paper presented to *IFS Seminar on Local Government Finance*, London, November.

LYOTARD, J-F. (1984) *The Postmodern Condition: A report on knowledge*, Manchester: Manchester University Press.

MAYNARD, A. (1994) 'Sickening effect of Surrey', *Health Service Journal*, 24 November, p. 19.

MAYNARD, A. and SHELDON, T.A. (1992) 'Reforming the Department of Health's research and development policy: from the devil to the deep blue sea', *British Medical Journal*, **305**(6863), pp. 1209–10.

PAGE, R. and DEAKIN, N. (Eds) (1993) *The Costs of Welfare*, Aldershot: Avebury.

PAHL, J. (1992) The impact of research on policy in social work and social welfare, in CARTER, P. and JEFFS, T. (Eds) *Changing Social Work and Welfare*, Buckingham: Open University Press.

PEARSON, G. (1983) *Hooligan. A History of Respectable Fears*, London: Macmillan.

POLLITT, C., HARRISON, S., HUNTER, D. and MARNOCH, G. (1990) 'No hiding place: on the discomforts of researching the contemporary policy process', *Journal of Social Policy*, **19**, pp. 169–90.

REPORT OF THE COMMISSION ON SOCIAL JUSTICE (1994) *Social Justice: Strategies for National Renewal*, London: Vintage.

ROTHSCHILD REPORT (1982) *An Enquiry into the Social Science Research Council*, Cmnd 8554, London: HMSO.

SCHUTZ, A. (1967) *The Phenomenology of the Social World*, Evanston IL: Northwestern University Press.

SMITH, G. (1994) *A Wider Strategy for Research and Development Relating to Personal Social Services*, Report to the Director of Research and Development: Department of Health.

SMITH, R. (1992) 'Audit and research', *British Medical Journal*, **307**, pp. 1403–7.

TAYLOR-GOOBY, P. (1994) 'Postmodernism and social policy: a great leap backwards', *Journal of Social Policy*, **23**(3), pp. 385–404.

TOURAINE, A. (1981) *The Voice and the Eye: An Analysis of Social Movements*, Cambridge: Cambridge University Press.

TULLOCK, G. (1965) *The Politics of Bureaucracy*, Washington D.C: Public Affairs Press.

VINCENT, J. (1992) 'Water under the bridge', in VINCENT, J. and BROWN, S. (Eds) *Critics and Customers: The Control of Social Policy Research*, Aldershot: Avebury.

WALKER, D. (1995) 'The rational anthem', *Times Higher Education Supplement*, February 17, pp. 15–16.

WALKER, R. (1989) 'We would like to know why: qualitative research and the policy – maker', *Research, Policy and Planning*, **7**(2), pp. 15–21.

WEBB, A. (1992) 'Funding social science research: nemesis of a new dawn', in VINCENT, J. and BROWN, S. (Eds) (1992) *Critics and Customers: The Control of Social Policy Research*, Aldershot: Avebury.

WICKS, M. (1987) 'Shaping the state', *Social Services Insight*, February 20 pp. 22–3.

WILLIAMS, F. (1992) 'Somewhere over the rainbow: Universality and diversity in social policy', in MANNING, N. and PAGE, R. (Eds) *Social Policy Review 4*, Canterbury: Social Policy Association.

WILLIAMS REPORT (1992) *Review of the Role of Department of Health Funded Research Units*, Report to the Director of Research and Development of a review team, London: Department of Health.

WOLLEN, P. (1993) *Raiding the Icebox: Reflections on Twentieth Century Culture*, London: Verso.

YOUNG, H. (1989) *One of Us: A Biography of Margaret Thatcher*, London: Macmillan.

Notes on Contributors

Karl Atkin is a senior research fellow in the Department of Social and Economic Studies, University of Bradford. His research interest is community care policy, and he has published on the experiences of carers, service organization and community care among people from black and ethnic minorities. He is joint-editor of *Race and Community Care* (Open University Press, 1996).

David Buck is a research fellow in the Centre for Health Economics, University of York. His current interests are in the economic analysis of health promotion and the economics of addictive substances.

Douglas Coyle was formerly a research fellow at the Centre for Health Economics. He is currently employed as a health economist at the Clinical Epidemiology Unit of the Ottawa Civic Hospital, University of Ottawa, Canada.

John Ditch is Professor of Social Policy at the University of York and Coordinator of the European Observatory on National Family Policies. Previously, he was Assistant Director of the Social Policy Research Unit where he was responsible for the social security research programme.

Tony Eardley is a senior research fellow at the Social Policy Research Centre in Sydney, Australia. Current research includes comparative studies of social security policy and he is part of the coordinating team for the European Observatory on National Family Policy. He is joint author of *Social Assistance Schemes in the OECD Countries* (HMSO, 1995) and *Low-Income Self-Employment: Work, Benefits and Living Standards* (Avebury, 1993).

Christine Godfrey is a senior research fellow at the Centre for Health Economics. Since 1984, she has been engaged in various research projects investigating economic aspects of alcohol, tobacco and other licit and illicit

198

drugs. She is co-editor of *Quality of Life: Perspectives and Policies* (Routledge, 1990) and *Preventing Alcohol and Tobacco Problems, Volume 2* (Avebury, 1990).

John Horton is reader in Political Theory at Keele University. He was formerly Director of the Morrell Studies in Toleration at the University of York. Recent publications include *Political Obligation* (Macmillan, 1993); he is joint editor of *After MacIntyre* (Polity, 1994) and *Literature and the Political Imagination* (Routledge, 1996).

Steven Kennedy is an information officer at the House of Lords. He was previously a research fellow at the Social Policy Research Unit where his research interests included comparative social policy, poverty and inequality, and tax, and benefit arrangements for older people and for families with children.

Jane Lightfoot is a research fellow in the Social Policy Research Unit. Her research interests include professional roles in community and primary health care, and needs assessment and accountability of professionals.

Neil Lunt is a research fellow in the Social Policy Research Unit. His research interests include community care policy and employment policy for disabled people.

Peter McLaverty was a research fellow in the Centre for Housing Policy, University of York. His research interests include housing benefit, tenant participation, and social theory and housing policy. He now lectures in Politics at the University of Luton.

Russell Mannion is a research fellow in the Centre for Health Economics. His research interests include community care policy, household finances and disability.

David Mayston is Professor of Public Sector Economics, Finance and Accountancy at the University of York. He is particularly interested in capital resource management and labour markets in health care, and issues of performance evaluation and expenditure in both health and education.

David Rhodes is a research fellow in the Centre for Housing Policy. His research interests include privately rented housing, housing benefit, and homelessness.

Gerald Richardson is a research fellow in the Centre for Health Economics. He has previously worked on the economics of alcohol taxation in the UK, the provision of services for alcohol and drug abusers by health and social agencies, and more generally on the cost-effectiveness of various treatments for substance misusers.

Roy Sainsbury is a senior research fellow in the Social Policy Research Unit. He has worked on projects on the computerization of the social security system, housing benefit, medical appeal tribunals, the implications of changing circumstances for benefit recipients, and benefits for disabled people.

Neil Small is a senior research fellow in both the Trent Palliative Care Centre and the University of Sheffield. His research interests concentrate on palliative care and on hospices. He is author of *Politics and Planning in the National Health Service* (Open University Press, 1989), and *AIDS, The Challenge: Understanding Education and Care* (Avebury, 1993).

Peter Smith is a reader in the Department of Economics and Related Studies at the University of York. His research interests are managerial efficiency and territorial allocation in the public sector.

Matthew Sutton is a research fellow in the Centre for Health Economics. His research interests include economic aspects of the consumption, supply and control of addictive substances.

Hilary Third was a research fellow in the Centre for Housing Policy, with interests in statutory and non-statutory homelessness, and voluntary sector agencies and homelessness. She is presently a research associate in the School of Planning and Housing at Heriot-Watt University.

Index

needs 71, 87, 143, 145, 147
    assessment 126–7, 129–33, 135
neo-classicalism 187–9
neo-conservatism 178
neo-liberalism 178–9
New, B. 123, 127, 135
New Economic Sociology 188–9
NHS
    community care 84–5, 91, 93
    professional accountability
        125–7
    racism 150
    Reforms 3–17
NHS and Community Care Act (1990)
    144, 151–2
Norman, A. 145, 152
nuclear family 63, 67, 74–5, 148
nursing homes 79–80, 87, 89

Oliver, M. 87, 101
opportunity, equality of 145–6, 151–2,
    154
owner occupation 37, 38, 42, 44

package care 78, 80, 87, 89
Parcel Force 5
Patel, Naina 146, 147
Patient's Charter 134
paying for community care 87
Pearson, G. 47, 48, 52, 181
Pearson, M. 145, 150
peer review 123, 127, 129, 136
pensions 88–9, 145, 164
performance of services 115, 117–18,
    121, 126
personal finance 87–9, 91–2, 94
Peters, B.G. 123, 124
pluralism 180, 187
political accountability 123–4, 126
political science 188–9
politics
    health care reform 4
    and ideas 178–9

Pollitt, C. 125, 126, 133–4, 135, 136,
    182
postmodernism 180–1, 190–3
poverty 60–1, 74, 92, 104, 145, 172
power 124–5, 132–3, 137, 146
pragmatism 180–1
Prescott-Clarke, P. *et al*. 35, 39
price of alcohol consumption 23–5,
    28–9, 32
primary care 84–5
priority setting 126–7, 130–3, 135–6
private
    health care 16
    housing 86
    rented sector 36–41
privatization 5, 9, 112, 114
professional accountability 123–8,
    131, 136–7
professional/manager 127, 132–7
professionalism 13, 98, 100–3
property
    benefits and 65, 67, 73
    community care and 89
    slump 42
providers 99–100, 112
    /purchasers 11, 13–14, 18, 78, 80,
        85, 91, 117, 126, 130–1, 133,
        144, 151, 183–6
public accountability 124, 126–7,
    134–7
public order disturbances 25
public services and market testing
    111–12, 115, 117–19, 121

qualitative analysis 176–7, 191–2
quality
    of community care 80
    measure of life 163–4
    of service 17, 111, 115–16, 119–21,
        125, 127, 129, 134, 136, 152
quantitative analysis 176–7, 192
Quintin, O. 170, 173